Acknowledgments

The U.S. Department of Health and Human Services (HHS) acknowledges:
Christine R. Dobday, Kimberly F. Stitzel, M.S., R.D., and Penelope Royall, P.T., M.S.W., with contributions from: Carter Blakey, Woodie Kessel, M.D., M.P.H., Barbara Schneeman, Ph.D., Camille Brewer, M.S., R.D., Kathleen Smith, M.S., R.D., Darla Danford, D.Sc., M.P.H., Eva Obarzanek, Ph.D., M.P.H., R.D., Janet M. de Jesus, M.S., R.D., Rebecca Payne, M.P.H., Harold W. Kohl, Ph.D., Melissa Johnson, M.S., Jane Wargo, M.A., Anne Hawthorn, Andrea Ducas, and Gloria Barnes, with the support of: Cristina Beato, M.D., and Laura Lawlor.

The Department also acknowledges the reviewers: Kathryn Y. McMurry, M.S., Mary Mazanec, M.D., J.D., Susan Merewitz, J.D., Laina Bush, M.B.A., Deb Galuska, Ph.D., Van Hubbard, M.D., Ph.D., Susan Anderson, M.S., R.D., Jean Pennington, Ph.D., R.D., Susan M. Krebs-Smith, Ph.D., R.D., William Dietz, M.D., Ph.D., Wendy Johnson-Taylor, Ph.D., Pamela Stark-Reed, Ph.D., Jennifer Seymour, Ph.D., Jean Lloyd, Ph.D., R.D., Yvonne Jackson, Ph.D., R.D., Jean Charles-Azure, M.P.H., R.D., Denise Sofka, M.S., R.D., Donna Robie, Ph.D., Steven Bradbard, Ph.D., Martina Vogel-Taylor, M.T., Christine Swanson, Ph.D., Deborah Nichols, M.D., Mary Kosinski, Meredith Terpeluk, Ira Dreyfuss, Jennifer Cabe, M.A., Wilma M. Tilson, M.P.H., and the USDA Dietary Guidance Work Group representatives.

The Department also acknowledges production assistance from: PSC/Visual Communications Branch, Porter Novelli, Daniel Morales, and Ginny Gunderson, with the support of the U.S. Government Printing Office.

Dietary Guidelines for Americans, 2005

The U.S. Department of Health and Human Services (HHS) and the U.S. Department of Agriculture (USDA) acknowledge the recommendations of the Dietary Guidelines Advisory Committee—the basis for this edition. The Committee consisted of Janet C. King, Ph.D., R.D. (chair), Lawrence J. Appel, M.D., M.P.H., Benjamin Caballero, M.D., Ph.D., Fergus M. Clydesdale, Ph.D., Penny M. Kris-Etherton, Ph.D., R.D., Theresa A. Nicklas, Dr.P.H., M.P.H., L.N., F. Xavier Pi-Sunyer, M.D., M.P.H., Yvonne L. Bronner, Sc.D., R.D., L.D., Carlos A. Camargo, M.D., Dr.P.H., Vay Liang W. Go, M.D., Joanne R. Lupton, Ph.D., Russell R. Pate, Ph.D., Connie M. Weaver, Ph.D., and the scientific writer/editor, Carol Suitor, Sc.D.

The Departments also acknowledge the work of the departmental scientists, staff, and policy officials responsible for the production of this document:

From HHS: Laura Lawlor, Michael O'Grady, Ph.D., Cristina Beato, M.D., Les Crawford, D.V.M., Ph.D., Barbara Schneeman, Ph.D., Kathryn Y. McMurry, M.S., Deb Galuska, Ph.D.,

Van Hubbard, M.D., Ph.D., Mary Mazanec, M.D., J.D., Penelope Royall, P.T., M.S.W., Laina Bush, M.B.A., Diane Thompson M.P.H., R.D., Susan Anderson, M.S., R.D., Jean Pennington, R.D., Ph.D., Susan M. Krebs-Smith, Ph.D., R.D., Wendy Johnson-Taylor, Ph.D., Kim Stitzel, M.S., R.D., Jennifer Weber, R.D., M.P.H., Pamela E. Starke-Reed, Ph.D., Paula R. Trumbo, Ph.D., Jennifer Seymour, Ph.D., Darla Danford, D.Sc., M.P.H, Christine Dobday, Donna Robie Howard, Ph.D., Ginny Gunderson, and Adam Michael Clark, Ph.D.

From USDA: Beth Johnson, M.S., R.D., Eric Bost, Eric Hentges, Ph.D., Kate Coler, Rodney Brown, Ph.D., Carole Davis, M.S., R.D., Dorothea K. Vafiadis, M.S., Joan M.G. Lyon, M.S., R.D., L.D., Trish Britten, Ph.D., Molly Kretsch, Ph.D., Pamela Pehrsson, Ph.D., Jan Stanton, M.S., M.B.A., R.D., Susan Welsh, Ph.D., Joanne Guthrie, M.P.H., R.D., Ph.D., David Klurfeld, Ph.D., Gerald F. Combs, Jr., Ph.D., Beverly Clevidence, Ph.D., Robert Mitchell Russell, M.D., Colette I. Thibault, M.S., R.D., L.D., Sedigheh-Essie Yamini, Ph.D., R.D., Kristin L. Marcoe, M.B.A., R.D., and David M. Herring, M.S.

The Departments also acknowledge the important role of those who provided input and public comments throughout this process. Finally, the Departments acknowledge the contributions of numerous other internal departmental scientists and staff that contributed to the production of this document, including the members of the Independent Scientific Review Panel who peer reviewed the recommendations of the document to ensure they were based on a preponderance of scientific evidence.

A Healthier You

Based on the Dietary Guidelines for Americans

U.S. Department of Health and Human Services

U.S. GOVERNMENT OFFICIAL EDITION NOTICE

Legal Status and Use of Seals and Logos

The seal of the U.S. Department of Health and Human Services (HHS) authenticates this publication as the Official U.S. Government edition of *A Healthier You*, a consumer handbook for use of the *Dietary Guidelines for Americans*, 2005, based upon a preponderance of scientific evidence and medical knowledge, pursuant to the mandates of Title III of the National Nutrition Monitoring and Related Research Act, Public Law 101-445.

Under the provisions of 42 U.S.C. 1320b-10, the unauthorized use of this seal in a publication is prohibited and subject to a civil penalty of up to $5,000 for each unauthorized copy of it that is reprinted or distributed.

HHS is the United States government's principal agency for protecting the health of all Americans and providing essential human services, especially for those who are least able to help themselves.

About ODPHP

The Office of Disease Prevention and Health Promotion (ODPHP), in the Office of Public Health and Science, provides leadership, coordination, and policy development for the disease prevention and health promotion priorities of HHS within the collaborative framework of the HHS agencies.

Use of ISBN Prefix

This is the Official U.S. Government edition of this publication and is herein identified to certify its authenticity. Use of the 0-16 ISBN prefix is for U.S. Government Printing Office Official Editions only. The Superintendent of Documents of the U.S. Government Printing Office requests that any reprinted edition be labeled clearly as a copy of the authentic work with a new ISBN.

2nd Printing

For sale by the Superintendent of Documents, U.S. Government Printing Office
Internet: bookstore.gpo.gov   Phone: toll free (866) 512-1800; DC area (202) 512-1800
Fax: (202) 512-2250   Mail: Stop SSOP, Washington, DC 20402-00001

ISBN 0-16-072525-9

DEPARTMENT OF HEALTH & HUMAN SERVICES   Public Health Service

Office of the Surgeon General
Rockville MD 20857

From the Nation's Doctor—Surgeon General, Dr. Richard H. Carmona

A Healthier Nation starts with a Healthier You.

One key to improving the health of our nation is to ensure individuals can access, understand, and use health-related information and services to make appropriate health decisions. Even the seemingly simple things we can do—such as eating healthy foods in healthy portions and being physically active every day—are sometimes difficult for us and our families. That is why the U.S. Department of Health and Human Services (HHS) developed this book for all Americans.

This book about healthy eating and physical activity is based on the *Dietary Guidelines for Americans (Dietary Guidelines)* and is full of practical, useful information.

A Healthier You brings together nutrition science and expertise to help Americans make smart choices from every food group, find balance between food and physical activity, and get the most out of the calories we consume.

A Healthier You is also a one-stop, easy-to-use resource for:
- science-based nutrition and physical activity guidance
- ways to use food labels to make smart purchase decisions
- healthy eating plans and worksheets to track your progress
- nearly 100 heart-healthy recipes
- helpful Web sites and tips.

Small, simple steps can often prevent or control chronic health problems such as diabetes, obesity, asthma, cancer, heart disease, and stroke. Prevention includes healthy eating habits and regular physical activity.

The choices you make about prevention are vital—for you and your family. Remember to help the children in your life learn healthy habits. Every day, when you interact with kids, you have an opportunity to be a role model. That is why there is a chapter in *A Healthier You* that is specific to children's needs.

It's great to develop healthy habits early in life, but it's also never too late to start. At any age, at every stage of life, everyone can make healthier choices.

As a doctor, too often I see that when someone has a health scare, he or she will change health habits for the better. But why wait until you get sick? Any time is a good time to start. You'll have the health benefits for the rest of your life!

Some of our unhealthy choices are the result of family traditions or convenience. Sometimes, we make unhealthy trade-offs because of what culture teaches us or because we're trying to save time in our busy lives.

Again, it's up to family leaders and community leaders to be role models…by eating healthy foods in healthy portions and by being physically active each day.

The *Dietary Guidelines* are for all of us.

These guidelines have a unique purpose in our nation. Federal nutrition programs are based on the *Dietary Guidelines*. And the *Dietary Guidelines* are not just one person's idea of science or health—they are the "state of the science."

Top scientists and health experts across our nation have studied the science and determined what works when it comes to nutrition and physical activity. Science is the heart and soul of the *Dietary Guidelines*.

As the United States Surgeon General, my job is to protect and advance the health of the nation. It's a tremendous responsibility to help improve the well-being of the American people.

Many Americans are living longer, primarily because of advances in technology. We want those years to be fulfilling, quality years. The reality is that better individual health will lead to stronger, healthier communities and a stronger nation.

Today, the United States spends more on health care than any other nation in the world. More than 125 million Americans live with chronic health problems. Chronic diseases, which are largely preventable through attention to healthy lifestyles—good nutrition, physical activity, preventive screenings, and making healthy choices—and preventive care, are factors in 70 percent of deaths each year and account for 75 percent of our $1.4 trillion in health care costs.

If current policies and conditions hold true, by the year 2011 our nation will spend over $2.8 trillion each year on health care.

That is one reason why HHS, in conjunction with the U.S. Department of Agriculture, developed the *Dietary Guidelines*.

A Healthier You is all about feeling better today and staying healthy for tomorrow. As a doctor, husband, parent, and public servant, I know firsthand that staying healthy is important to us in everything that we do and in everything that we can be.

Remember, the health of our nation begins…with a Healthier You.

Richard H. Carmona, M.D., M.P.H., F.A.C.S.
VADM, USPHS
United States Surgeon General

Table of Contents

A Healthier You
Based on the Dietary Guidelines for Americans

LIST OF FIGURES IN PART V

LIST OF TABLES IN PART V

Part I

Why Healthy Habits Matter— It's About You. For You.

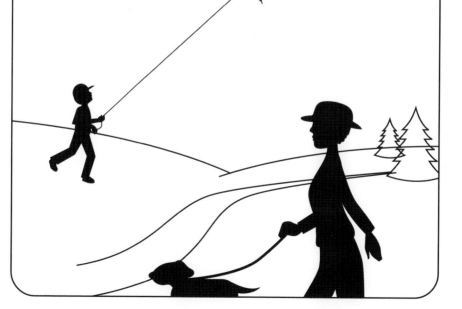

Chapter 1. Feel Better. Stay Healthy.

A Healthier You is all about feeling better today and staying healthy for tomorrow.

Ask yourself: "How do I feel? Am I as healthy as I can be—as I want to be every single day?" Doesn't it seem like the busier we get, the harder it is to make healthy choices—and stick to them?

We are bombarded with the latest studies or findings on what to eat, what not to eat, how much physical activity to get. Do these studies have merit? Are they trustworthy? What was good for us yesterday…isn't good for us today…and tomorrow, who knows? After a point, all of it seems more like noise than helpful news or information.

Despite the desire to tune it all out, that little voice inside us wants to pay attention because we really do want to be healthy! Don't we all

> ## **A HEALTHIER YOU**
>
> **We looked around America and saw people a lot like us. Some of us in shape. Many of us not. Some of us carrying too much around our middle— some of us carrying too much on our hips. Most of us not eating right. All of us, want- ing to know, what can we do about it? Not just about the weight but to be healthier.**
>
> **Together, let's find our way to a Healthier You!**

have the best intentions? The challenge is sorting through that conflicting, often- times confusing information from multiple sources or so-called experts. *A Healthier You* does just that. *A Healthier You* is not just one person's idea of science or what a diet should be. It reflects the thinking of top nutrition and health experts in the nation who have determined from the science what works. That information is in the *Dietary Guidelines for Americans*, which form the basis of this book and can be found in part V.

We also talked to people across the nation. We asked them what is important when it comes to their health—why is it important to be healthy? Virtually everyone agreed, "It's worth it because I want to be healthy for myself, my family…my future." We also talked about what scientists and nutritionists recommend for healthy eating and physical activity…and what information folks like you want. As you can imagine, we heard an earful. "Give me the basics," "…Not too much detail—or super technical stuff," while others said, "Not too little, I like in-depth information…" Everyone wants what's right for them—and, oh yeah, whatever it is has to work! But how do we know the information is reliable, proven, and right for us?

We asked ourselves, "What can we really do about this?" There's a lot. And, it's sensible—information that scientists and nutritionists agree on but that nobody has really pulled together in a way that everyone can understand and use. With that in mind, we set out to write *A Healthier You*. And, as Americans like you told us, "It's an investment in myself, and I have a say in what happens to me." We think that sums it up best. Reason enough to read on!

Chapter 2. Much More Than a Diet

A Healthier You is about our diet—what we eat. But it's not a "diet book." It's different. It's about helping us find our way to better health by making smart choices about nutrition and physical activity—two keys to a healthy lifestyle.

Sure, this raises a number of questions: "What exactly does a healthy lifestyle mean? Deny myself the very pleasures of eating? Is this the end of eating out? What about my hectic life? Seriously, how much physical activity do you really expect me to get each day?" Sometimes, it's hard enough to get everything done in a day—let alone physical activity!

A Healthier You is not about what we deny ourselves, but instead:

It's about choices. The food and physical activity choices we make every day affect our health. The more we know, the better choices we can make.

It's about balance. We need to learn to make more room in our lives for things that make us happy, healthy, and productive.

It's about a healthy lifestyle. To get the most out of our lives starts with small steps— a slow, steady approach to being healthy that we can live with each day—or most days. Hey, nobody's perfect!

At some level, we all know that a lot about being healthy comes down to taking care of ourselves: what we eat, how much we eat, and how much physical activity we get. We don't need to be rocket scientists to figure this out. *A Healthier You* already gives us the state of the science from the *Dietary Guidelines for Americans* to help us:
- make smart choices from every food group
- find our balance between food and physical activity
- get the most nutrition out of our calories.

Good to know, right? But let's face it, healthy habits take some effort. There's no magic pill that instantly does the trick.

How often have we told ourselves, "I'm going to start eating better and moving more." And, we mean it. We make the pact with ourselves at least every New Year. Too often, however, it's easy to get derailed and fall back into unhealthy habits. We don't mean to. But, the truth is—it takes a real commitment to change our behavior, especially for the long haul.

We basically know that we eat to live, but today, some of us seem to live to eat. Food represents a lot of things to us. To some it's a stress reducer—"I'm stressed. I'm tired and just want to go home and eat." There's often nothing like the emotional comfort of a pint of ice cream. Sometimes, food is our way of celebrating or a reason for coming together for special events like block parties or family reunions. Food is part of our social fabric. It's one way we pass traditions down from generation to generation and sometimes preserve our cultural identities. We hear stories from people talking about how food is part of their heritage. The secret ingredient in Nana's strudel is "love" to be sure, but there's also "lard" in that strudel! From Sunday family dinners serving spaghetti and meatballs to the best barbecue for a handful of nieces and nephews, extended family, and friends…sometimes, the entire neighborhood—we all love to kick back and relax with our favorite foods and enjoy ourselves!

There are ways, though, to make a healthier lifestyle doable and still enjoy Nana's cooking at the reunion. It's the day-in and day-out choices that we really need to think about. Whether this means finding the motivation to be our own personal trainer, using easy-to-make recipes to prepare our own meals in about as much time as it takes to head out to the nearest fast-food place, doing our best to eat healthfully on a budget, or making better choices when eating out—the little things do add up and make a big difference. Self-discipline may take some getting used to, so *A Healthier You* offers words not only of encouragement but also about the know-how to get started and keep with it!

Chapter 3. Being Healthy Matters to You

In the big picture, a number of things, in addition to food and physical activity, affect our health. Some of us struggle with reducing stress, getting enough sleep, or trying to quit smoking. Everyone is different. Today's decisions affect our health today, tomorrow, and beyond. Only we can figure out what is right for our lifestyle, but these decisions start with having the right information. That's where *A Healthier You* can help.

Healthy for life

It almost goes without saying that there are many benefits to improving our health. Developing good habits early in life helps, yet it's never too late to start. There is something to be said for starting to live a healthier life before gaining too much weight or becoming at risk for serious illness—to incorporate change while it's our decision. Why wait for a health scare to "get it together"? Wherever we are in life…whatever the reason…we can prevent many bad health consequences and gain quality time to enjoy things that really

> **Eating right and being physically active may reduce your risk for heart disease, high blood pressure, diabetes, osteoporosis, certain cancers, and being overweight or obese.**
>
> *Dietary Guidelines for Americans,* 2005

matter to us. Whether we are 15, 25, or 65, any time is a good time to start!

A lot of us have tried diets or started fitness programs. We stick with them for a while, then stop. The weight comes right back, or our cholesterol and blood pressure go back up.

> **Say to yourself, "This time it's going to be different—my efforts are going to result in a better, healthier me."**

Right now, wherever we are today, let's give ourselves a break. Make it a day to start with a clean slate. Our past choices are just that—past. Recognize that by taking small steps to eat better and be more physically active—even if we are starting from scratch—we can improve our health. And it doesn't take a lot to begin to have an impact.

"Me at my best"

We want to recapture that feeling—"me at my best." It's hard to describe, but you definitely know it when you feel it. People say, "When I'm eating healthy and being more active, it's like I'm energized" or "on top of my game!" Sometimes, don't you just dread the idea of taking time out for physical activity? Especially if it means getting out of bed a half hour earlier or squeezing it into a packed day. But afterwards, do you ever regret it? In fact, doesn't it change your mood for the rest of the day? It's empowering when you know you are taking control and making healthy changes that will make a difference for the rest of the day...the rest of your life. It's about looking and feeling better, knowing you are healthy inside and out. Wouldn't it be great to feel a renewed confidence in yourself or to simply take small steps to be your very best every day?

There's a lot of information about healthy living, but how do you find success for you—just for you? Take a moment. Think about what you want. You have a vision of who you want to be. Ask yourself, "What is 'me at my best'?" Write it down if you need to. Now, let's get started and find that healthier you...

Part II

Good Health Grounded in Science

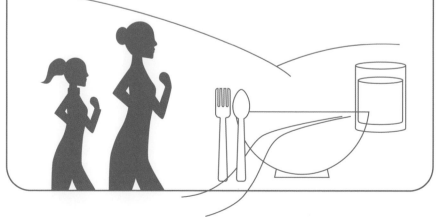

Chapter 4. Where to Start

It's official. Welcome to a Healthier You! Let's get started, but first things first.

Before you can begin making lifestyle changes and get on your way to a Healthier You, assess where you currently are. Ask yourself: "What is a healthy weight for me?" "How physically active am I?" "How many calories do I need?"

Personal Profile

This chapter will help answer these questions. You can write the answers to the questions on the worksheet, "My Personal Profile," on page 89. This will help you set goals and track your progress. You'll have different prompts after each question to let you know when to write information down in "My Personal Profile." That way, you will have all of your information in one place. To make it easy for you, tear out the worksheet in part III, "Making a Healthier You Happen"—that way you can copy them so every family member and friend has one. As you reach your goals, you will be able to see them and celebrate your successes together along the way!

On the other hand, along the way to a Healthier You, let's say you think you are not reaching your goals fast enough. You may begin to feel a little discouraged. By tracking your goals and progress, you'll have an opportunity to go back and review them, look at the changes you have been making, and begin to understand what obstacles may be blocking you from reaching your goals.

Human nature craves immediate results. Know this and be realistic in setting goals. You may need to make adjustments to how much you are eating, what kinds of foods you are eating, how much physical activity you are getting, or how much time you have allowed yourself to reach your goal.

For example, let's say your goal is to lose 10 pounds in 10 weeks. Typically, you measure your progress on a scale. Some weeks, you may lose 1 pound and some weeks you may even lose 2. Perhaps a week goes by and you don't see any weight loss. You start getting down on yourself and start doubting whether your plan works. Because you may be replacing fat with muscle and muscle weighs more than fat, you are not seeing the results you want on the scale. But, are your pants feeling a bit looser? Rest assured—you are making progress. The way your clothes fit may be a better measure than the scale from time to time. Even when your head tells you one thing, your body may be telling you something else. Give your body some time to adjust. Sometimes, it takes time for results to show on the outside—even if you may be making a difference on the inside.

Remember—we'll say this over and over again—this book is not a diet book, it's a lifestyle plan. *A Healthier You* shows the steps you can take to get you on your way.

Your healthy weight

Many Americans are overweight. Almost two-thirds of us are. Where do you fit in? It's fairly easy to tell. One common tool used as an indicator to determine whether you are at a healthy weight is the Body Mass Index, or BMI. Use the BMI chart below as an indication of your weight status—underweight, healthy weight, overweight, or obese. Locate your height in the left-most column, and read across the row from your height to your weight. Follow the column of the weight up to the top row that lists the BMI. A BMI of less than 19 is underweight, 19 through 24 is the healthy weight range, a BMI of 25 through 29 is the overweight range, and a BMI of 30 and above is the obese range.

Adult BMI Chart

BMI	19	20	21	22	23	24	25	26	27	28	29	30	31	32	33	34	35
Height							Weight in Pounds										
4'10"	91	96	100	105	110	115	119	124	129	134	138	143	148	153	158	162	167
4'11"	94	99	104	109	114	119	124	128	133	138	143	148	153	158	163	168	173
5'	97	102	107	112	118	123	128	133	138	143	148	153	158	163	158	174	179
5'1"	100	106	111	116	122	127	132	137	143	148	153	158	164	169	174	180	185
5'2"	104	109	115	120	126	131	136	142	147	153	158	164	169	175	180	186	191
5'3"	107	113	118	124	130	135	141	146	152	158	163	169	175	180	186	191	197
5'4"	110	116	122	128	134	140	145	151	157	163	169	174	180	186	192	197	204
5'5"	114	120	126	132	138	144	150	156	162	168	174	180	186	192	198	204	210
5'6"	118	124	130	136	142	148	155	161	167	173	179	186	192	198	204	210	216
5'7"	121	127	134	140	146	153	159	166	172	178	185	191	198	204	211	217	223
5'8"	125	131	138	144	151	158	164	171	177	184	190	197	203	210	216	223	230
5'9"	128	135	142	149	155	162	169	176	182	189	196	203	209	216	223	230	236
5'10"	132	139	146	153	160	167	174	181	188	195	202	209	216	222	229	236	243
5'11"	136	143	150	157	165	172	179	186	193	200	208	215	222	229	236	243	250
6'	140	147	154	162	169	177	184	191	199	206	213	221	228	235	242	250	258
6'1"	144	151	159	166	174	182	189	197	204	212	219	227	235	242	250	257	265
6'2'	148	155	163	171	179	186	194	202	210	218	225	233	241	249	256	264	272
6'3'	152	160	168	176	184	192	200	208	216	224	232	240	248	256	264	272	279
		Healthy Weight					Overweight					Obese					

Note: If your height or weight is not on this chart, please use the equation on page 89 to figure out your BMI.

Write down your current BMI in "My Personal Profile." Look at the BMI chart again and determine what a healthy weight range would be, based on your height. Write that down in "My Personal Profile," too. For example, if you are 5'7", your healthy weight could range between 121 and 153 pounds.

If you are underweight: If your BMI is less than 19, you may need to gain weight. If you do, use "My Healthy Eating Plan" to do so (more about this in chapter 7). And, don't forget to include physical activity. If you have recently lost 10 pounds or more without trying to lose weight, you may want to check with your health care professional.

If you are at a healthy weight: You may be at a "healthy weight," but not eating the right foods that give your body all the good nutrients you need to be healthy. For example, you may be at a healthy weight, but you may also not be eating enough fruits, vegetables, or whole grains. Being physically active is important even if you are at a healthy weight. This book is a starting point for finding your way to a Healthier You whatever your weight.

If you are at an unhealthy weight (obese or overweight): You should consider losing weight if you:
– are obese (BMI is greater than or equal to 30)
– are overweight (BMI of 25 to 29) and have two or more risk factors (see box)
OR
– have a high waist size (discussed on the next page) and two or more risk factors.
Modest weight loss (for example, 10 pounds) may have health benefits. Just as important is the prevention of further weight gain. Eating or drinking fewer calories while increasing physical activity are the keys to controlling body weight. Aim for slow, steady weight loss by eating fewer calories while getting the nutrients you need (that is, by maintaining an adequate intake of nutrients—the components of foods that affect your health). More details on this later, after you determine how physically active you are.

> **CHRONIC DISEASE RISK FACTORS**
> - High blood pressure (hypertension)
> - High LDL ("bad") cholesterol
> - Low HDL ("good") cholesterol
> - High triglycerides
> - High blood glucose (sugar)
> - Family history of premature heart disease
> - Cigarette smoking
> - Age (male ≥ 45 years, female ≥ 55 years)

If you are an athlete or muscular: The BMI chart may not be the best tool for you to determine your weight status. You may want to measure your waist size (see page 14) or to consult your health care provider to determine whether you are at a healthy weight.

Are you an apple or a pear? Extra fat in our belly area may put our health at risk, even if we are at a healthy weight. Men who have a waist size greater than 40 inches, and women who have a waist size greater than 35 inches, are at higher risk of diabetes, problems with cholesterol and triglycerides, high blood pressure, and heart disease because of excess abdominal fat. If your waist size is larger than these amounts, you should consider losing weight. Write your waist size in "My Personal Profile."

TO MEASURE YOUR WAIST SIZE

To measure your waist size (circumference), place a tape measure around your bare abdomen just above your hip bone. Be sure that the tape is snug, but does not compress your skin, and is parallel to the floor. Relax, exhale, and measure your waist.

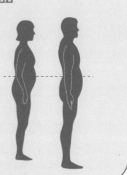

Remember: Eating right and being physically active aren't just a "diet" or a "program"—they are keys to a healthy lifestyle. With healthful habits, you may reduce your risk of many chronic diseases such as heart disease, diabetes, osteoporosis, and certain cancers, and may increase your chances for a longer life.

What about my kids? If you have children, you may be reading this book, to try to get helpful information for improving their lifestyle and nutrition. The BMI chart on page 12 should be used only to determine the weight status of adults. For kids, we use growth curve charts. Doctors use these to chart the height, weight, and age of children as they grow and develop. Chapter 12, "Healthier Children," will give you the information you need when talking to your kids about food and physical activity, and part IV, "Recipes and Resources," will help you make healthy choices when buying food and preparing meals.

Your healthy level of physical activity

So, now that you've determined whether or not you are at a healthy weight, how many calories are right for you? For now, we want to assess how many calories you need. A calorie is a scientific way to measure energy. You need to know about how physically active you are currently to estimate how many calories you need daily. Later on in the book, we'll discuss strategies for making small changes that will help you reach your healthy weight.

A Healthier You is about healthy eating **and** enough physical activity. The two go hand in hand. Regular physical activity is important for your overall health and fitness. Physical activity helps your body function, and it helps you control your body weight by burning up some of the calories you take in as food and beverages each day.

THE ENERGY BALANCE

CALORIES IN | CALORIES OUT

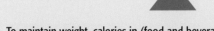

- To maintain weight, calories in (food and beverages consumed) should equal calories out (metabolism + routine activity + physical activity).
- To lose weight, calories in should be *less than* calories out.
- To gain weight, calories in should be *more than* calories out.

    Monitor weight: Over a few weeks, check your weight regularly, and adjust your calories in and out to stay on track with your goal.

How many calories are right for you?

What is my current physical activity level? You need to find out your physical activity level to determine your estimated daily calorie needs. Find out whether you are sedentary, moderately active, or active. Be honest with yourself. For the purposes of using the table on the next page to determine your calorie needs, we define sedentary, moderately active, and active as follows:

- *Sedentary* means a lifestyle that includes only the light physical activity associated with typical day-to-day life.
- *Moderately* active means a lifestyle that includes physical activity equivalent to walking about 1.5 to 3 miles per day at 3 to 4 miles per hour, in addition to the light physical activity associated with typical day-to-day life.
- *Active* means a lifestyle that includes physical activity equivalent to walking more than 3 miles per day at 3 to 4 miles per hour, in addition to the light physical activity associated with typical day-to-day life.

If you need more information, see chapter 10, "Making Physical Activity Part of a Healthier You."

Go to "My Personal Profile" on page 89, and fill out the section on your physical activity level.

Find your estimated daily calorie needs below. The calorie ranges shown are to accommodate needs of different ages within the age group.

For children and adolescents, more calories are needed at older ages. For example, a moderately active 13-year-old girl should aim for 2,000 calories, but a moderately active 9-year-old girl should aim for 1,600 calories.

For adults, fewer calories are needed at older ages. For example, an active 31-year-old man should aim for 3,000 calories, but an active 50-year-old man should aim for 2,800 calories.

		Activity Level		
		Sedentary	Moderately Active	Active
Gender	Age (years)	Calories		
Child	2–3	1,000	1,000–1,400	1,000–1,400
Female	4–8	1,200	1,400–1,600	1,400–1,800
	9–13	1,600	1,600–2,000	1,800–2,200
	14–18	1,800	2,000	2,400
	19–30	2,000	2,000–2,200	2,400
	31–50	1,800	2,000	2,200
	51+	1,600	1,800	2,000–2,200
Male	4–8	1,400	1,400–1,600	1,600–2,000
	9–13	1,800	1,800–2,200	2,000–2,600
	14–18	2,200	2,400–2,800	2,800–3,200
	19–30	2,400	2,600–2,800	3,000
	31–50	2,200	2,400–2,600	2,800–3,000
	51+	2,000	2,200–2,400	2,400–2,800

You have estimated the number of calories that you need each day based on your gender, age, and current physical activity. You are probably thinking to yourself, "If I am more active, I can eat more." But let's hold off on that concept for now. Right now, you are assessing your current habits—both food and physical activity. And you'll figure out what works for you and what changes you need to make to be a Healthier You.

Now, go to "My Personal Profile" on page 89, and write down your estimated calorie needs. At this point, you should have "My Personal Profile" filled in with your BMI, risk factors, physical activity level, healthy weight range, estimated daily calories, and goal. Below is a sample of a completed Personal Profile sheet:

My Personal Profile

Name: _Cindy_

Today's date: _January 2_

Age: _30_

Height (in.): _66 inches_

Weight (lb.): _170 pounds_   Waist size (in.): _36 inches_

BMI: Use the BMI chart on page 12 or use this equation:

$$\frac{wt\ (lb.)}{Height\ (in.)\ x\ height\ (in.)} \times 703 = \underline{\sim27}$$

BMI ranges:

- < 18.5 = underweight
- 18.5–24.9 = normal weight
- 25–29.9 = overweight
- > 30 = obese

My BMI indicates that I am: (Please circle)

underweight   normal weight   (overweight)   obese

My risk factors are: (Please circle)

- (high blood pressure) (hypertension)
- high LDL cholesterol ("bad" cholesterol)
- low HDL cholesterol ("good" cholesterol)
- high triglycerides

- high blood glucose (sugar)
- family history of premature heart disease
- (physical inactivity)
- cigarette smoking

My physical activity level is: (Please circle)

(sedentary)   moderately active   active

- *Sedentary* means a lifestyle that includes only the light physical activity associated with typical day-to-day life.
- *Moderately* active means a lifestyle that includes physical activity equivalent to walking about 1.5 to 3 miles per day at 3 to 4 miles per hour, in addition to the light physical activity associated with typical day-to-day life.
- *Active* means a lifestyle that includes physical activity equivalent to walking more than 3 miles per day at 3 to 4 miles per hour, in addition to the light physical activity associated with typical day-to-day life.

A healthy weight range for my height is: (Based on the BMI chart) _118-148 lbs_

Estimated daily calorie needs, my goal: _2,000_

Chapter 5. A Calorie Is a Calorie, or Is It?

We've been talking a lot about calories. Why? Because the number of calories you eat and drink, and use up through daily activities, is closely associated with your weight. Does it matter what types of foods the calories come from? Yes and no.

When it comes to calories and managing your weight, the answer is no. A calorie is a calorie is a calorie. Choosing healthy foods is important, and we'll address that in the next chapter, "Calories + Nutrients = Food." But first you need to learn about calories: what a calorie is, how to count calories, and how to set your calorie goal. This information will help you assess how close you are to your calorie goal. Then, you will be able to choose the kind of changes that will get you on your way to a Healthier You.

We know that most people don't like to count calories. It may feel like a daunting, overwhelming, and time-consuming task. We hear you. That is why *A Healthier You* is going to provide you with tools that will make it manageable for you to count calories and follow a healthy eating plan that you can make part of your everyday lifestyle.

What is a calorie?

A Calorie is the amount of heat needed to raise the temperature of a liter of water 1 degree. Sure, it was hard to understand when your science teacher explained it. Relax. It is just a scientific way to measure energy. That said, what do you need to know about calories? Just a few things: Think about what you regularly eat, what your calorie needs are, and how to count calories. It takes approximately 3,500 calories below your calorie needs to lose a pound of body fat. It takes approximately 3,500 calories above your calorie needs to gain a pound.

At this point, you know how many excess calories it takes to gain a pound or deficit calories to lose a pound (3,500), and you know about how many calories you need (in "My Personal Profile"). You are already on the road to a Healthier You! The next thing you need to learn is how to count calories so you can determine how many you eat each day. At first, this may seem like too much trouble, but once you get familiar with portion size and the number of calories in your favorite foods, you'll be able to estimate how many calories you eat each day, easily, without weighing your food and without taking too much of your valuable time.

ABOUT ANTHONY

Anthony is a 56-year-old man who is 5'10" and weighs 185 pounds. Anthony is a high school teacher and track coach who spends most of his day standing at work. Anthony does some light yard work when he returns home from work each day.

Using the BMI chart on page 12, Anthony determined that he has a BMI of 27. According to the BMI chart, he is overweight.

Next, using the definitions on page 15, Anthony determined his physical activity level. Because he does some physical activity while coaching and doing light yard work each day for at least 30 minutes, he is active.

Then, Anthony, using the calorie chart on page 16, determined his estimated calorie needs based on his age and current physical activity level. This is approximately 2,600 daily calories to maintain his current weight.

How many calories do you eat each day?

Calories count—and they come from both food and beverages. When eating packaged foods (for example, frozen, canned, and some prepared foods from the grocery store), counting your calories is easy—it's on the Nutrition Facts label. When eating foods that do not have a Nutrition Facts label, such as fresh fruits and vegetables, or when eating at home or in restaurants, determining calories is more difficult. If you can't count calories because there is no Nutrition Facts label, you should pay attention to portion size.

Use the Nutrition Facts label. Most packaged foods have a Nutrition Facts label. An example of one is on the next page. You can use this tool to make smart food choices and to find out how many calories and nutrients you are actually eating. To use the label effectively to count calories, you need to *check serving size, servings per container, and calories*. Look at the serving size and the number of servings per container. How many servings are you consuming? If you are eating 2 servings, you are eating double the calories and the nutrients listed on the Nutrition Facts label.

Portion size is the amount of food eaten at one time. Serving size is the amount stated on the Nutrition Facts label. Sometimes, the portion size and serving size match; sometimes, they don't. For example, if the label says that 1 serving size is 6 cookies and you eat 3, you've eaten ½ of a serving of cookies. More importantly, you have just reduced by half the calories listed on the Nutrition Facts label. Remember that the serving size on the Nutrition Facts label is not a recommended amount to eat; it's a simple and easy way for letting you know the calories and nutrients in a certain amount of a food. If the label helps you be more aware of how much you eat or drink—all the better!

When eating foods without a Nutrition Facts label, pay attention to how your portion size compares to a recommended amount of food from each food group. In chapter 7, "Breaking It Down," we'll show you how to do this.

Some foods prepared at the grocery store and other foods such as produce items may not have food packaging that provides nutritional information, but this information can sometimes be obtained in the store by request. Many restaurants have nutrition information on the foods they serve available at the restaurant or on their Web site. As grocery stores increase the number of prepared products that have nutrition information, it will become easier for you to make lower-calorie choices to help you control your calories every day. Don't be afraid to ask for nutrition information if you don't see it displayed at the grocery store or on the menu when eating out.

Nutrition Facts

Serving Size 1 cup (228g)
Servings Per Container 2

Amount Per Serving

Calories 260   Calories from Fat 120

	% Daily Value*
Total Fat 13g	**20%**
Saturated Fat 5g	**25%**
Trans Fat 2g	
Cholesterol 30mg	**10%**
Sodium 660mg	**28%**
Total Carbohydrate 31g	**10%**
Dietary Fiber 0g	**0%**
Sugars 5g	
Protein 5g	

Vitamin A 4%	•	Vitamin C 2%
Calcium 15%	•	Iron 4%

* Percent Daily Values are based on a 2,000 calorie diet. Your Daily Values may be higher or lower depending on your calorie needs:

	Calories:	2,000	2,500
Total Fat	Less than	65g	80g
Sat Fat	Less than	20g	25g
Cholesterol	Less than	300mg	300mg
Sodium	Less than	2,400mg	2,400mg
Total Carbohydrate		300g	375g
Dietary Fiber		25g	30g

Calories per gram:
Fat 9 • Carbohydrate 4 • Protein 4

On the sample Nutrition Facts label above, the serving size of this food is 1 cup, and there are 2 servings in this container. There are 260 calories per serving of this food. If you eat the entire container of this product, you will eat 2 servings. That means you need to double the calories (260 calories x 2 = 520 calories) to know how many calories you are eating. If you eat 2 servings, you will have eaten over 500 calories!

Now, you've learned how to use food packaging to help you figure out how many calories you are eating. In the following chapter, you will learn how to build healthy eating patterns using food groups. Estimating how many calories you are getting from these foods can be challenging at first. But since one of the best ways to manage your weight is to be aware of foods and beverages high in calories, being able to keep track of where your calories are coming from is an important skill that will help you for the rest of your life.

Setting your calorie goal

In chapter 4, "Where to Start," you determined your Body Mass Index, or BMI, to assess whether you were underweight, at a healthy weight, overweight, or obese. Staying at—or getting to—a healthy weight can help us in several ways. Not only might it help us feel better and look better, but science shows it plays an important role in reducing our risk of several types of chronic diseases that can definitely interfere with our hopes for a long, healthy life.

Excess body fat leads to a higher risk for premature death, type 2 diabetes, high blood pressure, problems with cholesterol and triglycerides, heart disease, stroke, gallbladder disease, lung problems, gout, arthritis, and certain kinds of cancers.

Dietary Guidelines for Americans, 2005

There is a right number of calories for you. This number depends on your age, gender, weight, activity level, and whether you're trying to gain, maintain, or lose weight. In chapter 4, "Where to Start," you estimated how many calories you need to maintain your weight at your current physical activity level.

If you are at a healthy weight (BMI between 19 and 24), then use the number of calories you estimated as your calorie needs based on your current physical activity level. This is the number you wrote down in "My Personal Profile." In chapters 9 and 10, you will determine whether you are physically active enough to reduce your risk for developing a chronic disease or to maintain or achieve a healthy weight.

If you are obese, overweight, or have a high waist size and two or more risk factors (see page 13), even modest weight loss (for example, 10 pounds) has health benefits. Preventing further weight gain is very important. Eating fewer calories while increasing physical activity are the keys to controlling body weight. Simply put, eat less, move more. If you need to lose weight, aim for slow, steady weight loss by decreasing calorie intake while maintaining an adequate intake of nutrients. Next are a couple of suggestions to get you on your way.

If you need to lose weight, a reduction of 500 or more calories each day from added sugar, fat, and alcohol is a good strategy. For example, drink water flavored with lemon or lime, seltzer water, or a diet soda instead of a sugar-sweetened beverage, or use a non-caloric sweetener instead of a sweetener with calories. Together these small changes can quickly add up to 500 calories! Later on, we will give you more details on how to do this.

tip
for controlling calories:

On the Nutrition Facts label, when 1 serving of a single food item contains 400 or more calories, it's high; and 40 calories is low.[1]

The packaging of a food can also contain other useful information for making your food selections. For example, sometimes, foods are labeled "calorie free," "low calorie," "reduced or lower in calories," "light," or "lite." Here is a quick guide to what those words mean:

Calorie free = Less than 5 calories per serving.

Low calorie = 40 calories or less per serving.

Reduced calorie or lower in calories = At least 25 percent fewer calories than the regular version.

Light or lite = Half the fat or a third of the calories of the regular version.[2]

[1] Based on 2,000 calories.
[2] For example, if a regular cheesecake has 300 calories and 8 grams of fat per serving, then the "lite" version could have 200 calories and 4 grams of fat per serving.

Chapter 6. Calories + Nutrients = Food

In this chapter, we'll talk about why the types of foods your calories come from matter. Calories plus nutrients equals food…well, there is more to it than that. But the important thing to know is when you eat and drink, you take in nutrients and calories.

Now that you have a goal for **how many calories** you need to achieve or maintain a healthy weight (you wrote it in "My Personal Profile"), it is time to learn **what types and amounts** of foods to eat that will be healthy, satisfying, and meet your calorie goal. You may be eating enough food, but not eating the right foods that give your body the nutrients you need to be healthy. What you eat is just as important as how much you eat. A healthy eating plan is one that:

- Emphasizes fruits, vegetables, whole grains, and fat-free or low-fat milk and equivalent milk products. Specifically, many fruits and vegetables are packed with nutrients but have very few calories.
- Includes lean meats, poultry, fish, beans (legumes), eggs, and nuts.
- Is low in saturated and *trans* fats, cholesterol, salt (sodium), and added sugars.
- Balances calorie intake with calorie needs.

Let's talk about why healthy eating is important.

What are nutrients?

Nutrients are substances that play a role in health. For example, vitamins and minerals are nutrients, as are fats, protein, and carbohydrates. Nutrients are in foods and can come from dietary supplements. However, the *Dietary Guidelines for Americans*, the basis for this book, makes a point that nutrients consumed should come primarily from foods. Foods contain vitamins and minerals that are often found in supplements, but food also contains hundreds of beneficial naturally occurring substances that may protect against chronic health problems. Therefore, if you have a choice between an orange or a vitamin C supplement, it is better to eat the orange.

Some specific groups of people have higher requirements for certain nutrients and may benefit from use of vitamin and mineral supplements. These groups include women of childbearing age, who may become pregnant; women who are in their first trimester (that is, the first 3 months) of pregnancy; people over 50; people with dark skin; and people who don't get enough sunlight. If you fall into one of these groups, we have more specifics for you on pages 262 to 263, in part V. However, most people will not need to exceed 100% of their RDA. RDA stands for Recommended Dietary Allowance—the amount of a specific nutrient needed each day.

Why are nutrients important for you?

It is important that you meet your recommended nutrient needs because they offer important benefits—normal growth and development of children, health promotion for people of all ages, and reduction of risk for a number of chronic diseases.

In part V, "Dietary Guidelines for Americans, 2005," there is a thorough discussion regarding the health benefits of consuming specific nutrients. We encourage you to read it. But for those of you who want to know what to do without more of the why, you can start here. For the rest of you who want to know more of the why and the science behind the why, pages 257 to 264, in part V, are for you.

Many Americans don't consume the right amount of many nutrients. For each of us, there is a recommended need for specific nutrients. This need is based on our age and gender. From data collected by the federal government and scientists across the nation, we know the nutrients Americans need to pay special attention to, because they may not be getting enough of them:

- **Adults:** calcium, potassium, fiber, magnesium, and vitamins A, C, and E
- **Children and adolescents:** calcium, potassium, fiber, magnesium, and vitamin E
- **Specific population groups:** vitamin B_{12}, iron, folic acid, and vitamins E and D

For example, women of childbearing age, who may become pregnant, and women who are in their first trimester (that is, the first 3 months) of pregnancy need to pay attention to their folic acid intake. Also, adolescents, women of childbearing age, who may become pregnant, and pregnant women (at all stages) need to watch their iron intake.

Maximizing your nutrients—making calories work for you

The main premise of this book is that food should provide you with all the nutrients you need for growth and health. You may be saying to yourself, "How am I going to control my calories and get enough nutrients? This is too much information."

Earlier, you set your calorie goal and learned how to monitor your intake. Calories are one aspect of your diet. Another is trying to eat types and amounts of food that will promote health and help prevent chronic diseases. You could use up all of your calories on a few high-calorie foods or drinks, but if you did, chances are you wouldn't get the full range of nutrients your body needs to be healthy. Choose the most nutritionally rich foods you can each day—those packed with vitamins, minerals, fiber, and other nutrients but lower in calories. Pick foods like fruits, vegetables, dry beans and peas, whole grains, and fat-free or low-fat milk and equivalent milk products more often.

At first, this may seem like a lot of information. You don't have to do everything at once. Remember, this is a lifestyle makeover, not quick weight loss. Relax. You can pick one aspect of your diet to work on at a time. We want to help you find what works for you. In the following chapters, you will find tips and resources to help you set goals for yourself.

Chapter 7. Breaking It Down

Now, you are going to learn what makes up a healthy eating plan and the amounts of each food group necessary to meet your nutrient and calorie needs. A warning: this chapter is a little long, and it is packed full of information. But, there is light at the end of the tunnel. If you need to, go through this chapter a little at a time—in bite-size pieces. The payoff is big. At the end, you will have a healthy eating plan, full of foods you already like, designed by you. Are you excited? We are.

What is a healthy eating plan?

In chapter 6, "Calories + Nutrients = Food," we learned a healthy eating plan is one that:

- Emphasizes fruits, vegetables, whole grains, and fat-free or low-fat milk and equivalent milk products. Specifically, many fruits and vegetables are packed with nutrients but have few calories.
- Includes lean meats, poultry, fish, beans (legumes), eggs, and nuts.
- Is low in saturated and *trans* fats, cholesterol, salt (sodium), and added sugars.
- Balances calorie intake with calorie needs.

...and tastes good too!

So, what does this mean? In this book, appendix A has examples of two healthy eating plans, the Dietary Approaches to Stop Hypertension (DASH) Eating Plan[1] and the USDA Food Guide.[2] We will use the DASH Eating Plan as an example. From this, you can map out how much you need from each food group based on your calorie needs.

What are the food groups?

The food groups we are referring to categorize foods into major groups:

- Grains
- Fruits
- Vegetables
- Milk and milk products
- Meats, poultry, and fish
- Nuts, seeds, and legumes

Sometimes, meat, poultry, and fish, and nuts, seeds, and legumes, are referred to as the "protein group."

---

[1] This eating plan was originally developed and studied by scientists at the National Institutes of Health to lower blood pressure. But it is much more than that. It meets all of your recommended nutrients within your calorie needs and allows you the flexibility to enjoy healthful foods. For more detailed information about the DASH Eating Plan, please visit www.nhlbi.nih.gov.

 [2] You can find detailed information about the USDA Food Guide, better known as MyPyramid, on its Web site: www.mypyramid.gov. This Web site provides a personalized food intake pattern based on your age, gender, and physical activity level, as well as the MyPyramid Tracker, an interactive diet and activity assessment tool.

My Healthy Eating Plan

Let's get started on filling out a healthy eating plan for you. This will be your goal to strive for when eating healthfully. Once you've completed "My Healthy Eating Plan," you'll have an eating plan that is relevant to and realistic for you, because it will be full of food you like. Remember, this is about you, and what works for you.

In chapter 5, "A Calorie Is a Calorie, or Is It?"—you set your calorie goal. Now, you use your calorie goal, and we'll use our friend Jennifer as an example to illustrate how a completed plan looks. You can use either plan in appendix A that works for you (DASH Eating Plan or USDA Food Guide). For this example, Jennifer used the 2,000-calorie level of the DASH Eating Plan to determine what and how much she should eat from each food group. Jennifer's calorie goal is 2,000 calories. She filled out her plan for each food group.

Now, it's your turn. Turn to page 91, "My Healthy Eating Plan." Write in your calorie goal. Next, use the information in appendix A, on page 320, to fill in how much from each food group you can eat each day. Write the number of daily servings of each food group in the food group boxes at the top of "My Healthy Eating Plan." Is it more or less than Jennifer needs to eat?

ABOUT JENNIFER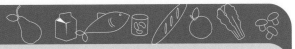

Jennifer is a 30-year-old female who is 5'5" and weighs 125 pounds. She is a computer specialist who spends most of her day at her desk at work. She walks a mile to and from work each day.

Using the BMI chart on page 12, Jennifer determined that she has a BMI of approximately 21. According to the BMI chart, she is at a healthy weight.

Next, using the definitions on page 15, Jennifer determined her physical activity level. Her activity level is equivalent to 2 miles per day. She is moderately active.

Then, using the calorie chart on page 16, Jennifer estimated her calorie needs based on her age and current physical activity level. Jennifer's calorie needs are approximately 2,000 daily calories.

Next, we are going to tell you in detail what we mean by food groups, what you need to eat in each of the food groups and why, and how to meet your goal for consuming a healthy diet. We also have tips on how to get these healthy foods into your daily eating plan whether you are getting your food at the grocery store, at home, or on the go.

First look at this table, which shows you the food groups, the number of servings in each group needed for a 2,000-calorie diet, and a few examples of foods that equal 1 serving.

Food Groups	2,000-Calorie Eating Plan	Serving Sizes (1 serving)
Grains[a]	6–8 servings	1 slice bread 1 oz dry cereal[b] 1/2 cup cooked rice, pasta, or cereal
Vegetables	4–5 servings	1 cup raw leafy vegetable 1/2 cup cut-up raw or cooked vegetable 1/2 cup vegetable juice
Fruits	4–5 servings	1/2 cup fruit juice 1 medium fruit 1/4 cup dried fruit 1/2 cup fresh, frozen, or canned fruit
Fat-free or low-fat milk and equivalent milk products	2–3 servings	1 cup fat-free or low-fat milk 1 cup fat-free or low-fat yogurt 1 1/2 oz fat-free, low-fat, or reduced fat cheese
Lean meats, poultry, and fish	2 or less servings	3 oz cooked meat, poultry, or fish (1 oz meat = 1 egg[c])
Nuts, seeds, and legumes	4–5 servings per week	1/3 cup or 1 1/2 oz nuts 2 Tbsp peanut butter 2 Tbsp or 1/2 oz seeds 1/2 cup cooked dry beans or peas

[a] Whole grains are recommended for most grain servings to meet fiber recommendations.

[b] Equals 1/2 to 1 1/4 cups, depending on cereal type. Check the product's Nutrition Facts label.

c Since eggs are high in cholesterol, limit egg yolk intake to no more than 4 per week because of the saturated fat and cholesterol content; two egg whites have the same protein content as 1 oz of meat.

The number of servings is per day unless otherwise stated.

Now, let's talk more in depth about why each food group is important for your health, assess how much of each food group you currently eat, and set goals for what you need to eat to be a Healthier You. You may notice that fats and oils, and sweets, on "My Healthy Eating Plan" are not in the table. We'll talk about them in the next chapter.

Eat fruits and vegetables.

You've probably heard this all of your life—fruits and vegetables are good for you, and it's important to eat them every day.

It may help to know why.

Fruits and vegetables may reduce the risk of several chronic diseases. Compared to people who don't eat enough fruits and vegetables, people who eat them daily as part of a healthy diet are likely to have reduced risk of chronic diseases, including stroke and perhaps other cardiovascular diseases, type 2 diabetes, and cancers in certain parts of the body (mouth, throat, lung, esophagus, stomach, and colon-rectum).

A healthy diet is one that: emphasizes a variety of fruits, vegetables, whole grains, and fat-free or low-fat milk and equivalent milk products; includes lean meat, poultry, fish, legumes (dry beans and peas), eggs, nuts, and seeds; and balances calorie intake with calorie needs. Sound familiar?

The fiber in fruits, vegetables, and legumes is important. Healthful diets rich in fiber-containing foods may reduce the risk of heart disease. In addition to fiber, many fruits and vegetables are also rich in other nutrients such as vitamins A and C, folate, and potassium—which are important because many of us don't eat enough foods with these nutrients. **And, these nutrients are particularly important for women who are or may become pregnant.**[3] In chapter 6, "Calories + Nutrients = Food," we discussed nutrients and their role in reducing risks for chronic diseases and promoting health. On the next page is a short list for your reference when you are looking for ideas to get more fruits and vegetables into your diet. A more extensive list for each of these nutrients is in appendix B,[4] beginning on page 328.

Eating fruits and vegetables provides other benefits, too. One is calorie control. Many fruits and vegetables are low in calories and packed with nutrients or "nutrient dense"—a term that is gaining popularity in the "diet world." So, if you're trying to lose weight, fruits and vegetables can help you feel full. Fruits and vegetables are

[3] Since folic acid reduces the risk of the neural tube defects, spina bifida, and anencephaly in the developing fetus, a daily intake of 400 ug/day of synthetic folic acid (from fortified foods or supplements in addition to food forms of folate from a varied diet) is recommended for women of childbearing age who may become pregnant. Folic acid is critical for fetal development, especially before the woman knows she is pregnant. Pregnant women should consume 600 ug/day of synthetic folic acid (from fortified foods or supplements) in addition to food forms of folate from a varied diet. It is not known whether the same level of protection could be achieved by using food that is naturally rich in folate.

[4] Appendix B contains food sources of selected nutrients: potassium, vitamin E, iron, non-dairy sources of calcium, calcium, vitamin A, magnesium, dietary fiber, and vitamin C.

packed with vitamins, minerals, fiber, and other important nutrients—have we made that point yet? They can help you get the most nutrition out of the daily number of calories you're supposed to eat for a Healthier You. Remember, different fruits and vegetables are rich in different nutrients, so aim for a variety. And when eating vegetables, include those that are dark green and leafy or orange, and don't forget dry beans and peas.

How many fruits and vegetables do you need?

Look at "My Healthy Eating Plan." How many fruits and vegetables do you need each day? How does this number compare with what you usually eat each day? Let's look at Jennifer's eating plan on the next page. In it, we've italicized the foods that we are talking about. You will see this eating plan throughout this chapter. Jennifer will make minor adjustments to it as she develops her healthy eating plan.

Nutrients in Fruits and Vegetables	
Sources of vitamin A • Bright orange vegetables like carrots, sweet potatoes, and pumpkin • Tomatoes and tomato products, and red sweet pepper • Leafy greens such as spinach, collards, turnip greens, kale, beet and mustard greens, green leaf lettuce, and romaine • Orange fruits like mangoes, cantaloupe, apricots, and red or pink grapefruit	**Sources of folate** • Cooked dry beans and peas • Oranges and orange juice • Deep green leaves like spinach and mustard greens
Sources of vitamin C • Citrus fruits and juices, kiwi fruit, strawberries, guava, papaya, and cantaloupe • Broccoli, peppers, tomatoes, cabbage (especially Chinese cabbage), Brussels sprouts, and potatoes • Leafy greens such as romaine, turnip greens, and spinach	**Sources of potassium** • Baked white or sweet potatoes, cooked greens (such as spinach), and winter (orange) squash • Bananas, plantains, many dried fruits, oranges and orange juice, cantaloupe, and honeydew melons • Cooked dry beans • Soybeans (green and mature) • Tomato products (sauce, paste, and purée) • Beet greens

ABOUT JENNIFER

Jennifer should be eating 8 to 10 servings of fruits and vegetables each day (4 to 5 servings of fruits and 4 to 5 servings of vegetables) based on her calorie needs (2,000 calories). That is about 2 cups of fruit and 2 cups of vegetables. She figured out how to spread this out throughout the day. First, she asked herself what fruits she likes. Then, she asked herself what vegetables she likes. She wrote down the following:

Favorite fruits: bananas, apples, nectarines, plums, canned peaches, orange juice, strawberries, raspberries, and oranges
Favorite vegetables: lettuce, spinach, potatoes, tomato sauce, green beans, carrots, and corn

Next, Jennifer figured out how she could plan to eat these foods through-out the day. She usually eats lunch with her co-workers; they often get sandwiches for lunch. She's planned on having pasta and bean salad for dinner and raspberries for dessert. Knowing that, Jennifer realized that she needed to get in about 1 1/2 cups of fruit throughout the day, since she plans to get her vegetables and some fruit at home that evening. Jennifer decided she would try to eat the following foods during the day:
Breakfast: *medium banana*, fat-free peach yogurt, and coffee with fat-free milk
Lunch: turkey, with whole wheat roll; *romaine lettuce, tomato, and cucumber*, with light Italian dressing; *medium orange*; and unsweetened iced tea
Dinner: pasta and bean salad (1 cup whole wheat pasta, 1/2 cup chick-peas, *1 cup chopped vegetables [carrots, green peppers, and onions]*, with olive oil) and 1 cup of fat-free milk
Dessert: *raspberries (1 cup)*

Jennifer checked her fruits and vegetables to make sure she has a variety of different kinds.

Now, it's your turn. Write down the fruits you like, in the space on the next page. If you need any ideas, look at the different lists of food sources of nutrients in appendix B.

Fruits I like:

_____

_____

_____

_____

Now, write down the vegetables you like, in the space below. You can use appendix B again if you need some help thinking of vegetables.

Vegetables I like:

_____

_____

_____

_____

What if I don't like fruits and vegetables?

Some of us think we don't like fruits and vegetables. But maybe we don't like what we've tried. Look at the list of foods in appendix B and try something you've never tried before—or try them in another form. For example, if you've tried canned carrots and didn't like them, try them raw with a low-fat hummus dip or salsa.

Now, write down when you could eat these fruits and vegetables throughout the day. Try to make sure you choose a variety.

Breakfast:

_____

Lunch:

_____

Dinner:

_____

Snack:

_____

Dessert:

_____

One way to make it easier to eat fruits and vegetables is to keep them stocked at home and ready to eat when you get hungry. So, let's go shopping!

At the grocery store. You can buy fruits and vegetables canned, frozen, dried, or fresh. There is a sample grocery shopping list in part III, "Making a Healthier You Happen," to help you pick up these healthy treats at the grocery store.

When shopping for fruits and vegetables, choose an assortment of different types and colors to provide you with a variety of nutrients. Buy fruits and vegetables you are most likely to eat, and sometimes, try something new! It is fun to try fruits and vegetables you haven't tried before; you may find that you can add another favorite to your list. Remember, if you buy fresh fruits and vegetables, buy only what you will eat that week, because fresh fruits and vegetables can spoil.

A good way to save money and make sure you always have fruits and vegetables in your home is to stock up on packaged (canned, frozen, and dried) fruits and vegetables. For additional money-saving tips, we have a list in part IV, "Recipes and Resources."

One caution about buying canned, frozen, or dried fruits or vegetables: they may contain added sugars, saturated fats, or sodium—ingredients you may want to limit. There are three places to look on a package that give you clues to what is in the food: the ingredient list, the Nutrition Facts label, and the front label of the package. Added sugars can appear on the **ingredient list** as brown sugar, sucrose, glucose, dextrose, high fructose corn syrup, invert sugar syrup, corn syrup, maple syrup, honey, and fructose. A more extensive list is on page 304.

This sample product ingredient list for frozen sweetened strawberries shows you that it contains added sugars.

INGREDIENTS: Strawberries, invert sugar syrup, corn syrup.

For canned, dried, or frozen fruits and vegetables, use the Nutrition Facts label to check the calories, serving size, nutrient content, and percent Daily Value (% DV).[5] Compare similar products and make sure the serving sizes are comparable. To make your calories count, compare the calories and % DV for the nutrients you want to limit or get enough of per serving size.

---

[5] The % DVs are based on the Daily Value recommendations for key nutrients for a 2,000-calorie diet. Whether or not you consume more or less than 2,000 calories, you can use the % DV to help you determine whether the food or drink is high or low in a nutrient for the serving size listed on the Nutrition Facts label.

To help make your decisions faster, use the Nutrition Facts label on many food packages. A quick guide to using the % DV: 5% DV or less is low, and 20% DV or more is high. You should keep saturated fat, *trans* fat, cholesterol and sodium as low as possible and get enough of other nutrients such as potassium, fiber, vitamins A and C, calcium, and iron.

While fruits and vegetables are rich in nutrients, you need to remember that packaged fruits and vegetables may contain added fat, salt (sodium), and sugars that can increase those nutrients you want less of. So, to be safe, always use the Nutrition Facts label. We'll discuss more about the Nutrition Facts label throughout the book.

Nutrition Facts

Serving Size 1 cup (228g)
Servings Per Container 2

Amount Per Serving		
Calories 250	Calories from Fat 110	
		% Daily Value*
Total Fat 12g		18%
Saturated Fat 3g		15%
Trans Fat 3g		
Cholesterol 30mg		10%
Sodium 470mg		20%
Potassium 700mg		20%
Total Carbohydrate 31g		10%
Dietary Fiber 0g		0%
Sugars 5g		
Protein 5g		
Vitamin A		4%
Vitamin C		2%
Calcium		20%
Iron		4%

Check calories

Quick guide to % DV

5% or less is low
20% or more is high

Limit these

Get enough of these

* Percent Daily Values are based on a 2,000 calorie diet. Your Daily Values may be higher or lower depending on your calorie needs.

	Calories:	2,000	2,500
Total Fat	Less than	65g	80g
Sat Fat	Less than	20g	25g
Cholesterol	Less than	300mg	300mg
Sodium	Less than	2,400mg	2,400mg
Total Carbohydrate		300g	375g
Dietary Fiber		25g	30g

SOUND BITES:

- At the beginning of a meal, ask yourself how many fruits and vegetables you've eaten that day. Then, try to add one or two fruits or vegetables if you still haven't met your goal.
- If fruits and vegetables are canned, dried, or frozen, read the label and avoid those with saturated fat, added salt (sodium), and added sugars.
- When you're increasing the amounts of fruits and vegetables you eat, eat them *instead of* less nutritious foods.
- Put fruits and vegetables on your shopping list—choose an assortment of different types and colors to provide you with a variety of nutrients.
- When eating at a restaurant, order a low-fat vegetable dish as an appetizer or salad. Order fruit as a dessert. Watch out for added fat or sugar!

In addition, **the label on the front of the package** may contain statements or claims about the product made by the food manufacturer. Use the claims on fruit and vegetable packages to identify foods with little salt (sodium) or added sugars. Examples include "low sodium," "no salt added," "no added sugar," and "unsweetened."

Eat calcium-rich foods.

Another source of important nutrients is milk and milk products like fat-free or low-fat yogurt and cheese. Consuming milk products is especially important to bone health during childhood and adolescence—but it is also important at anytime in our lives. Diets rich in milk and milk products may reduce the risk of weakened bones throughout your lifetime. Adults and children should not avoid milk and milk products because of concerns that these foods lead to weight gain. Many fat-free and low-fat choices without added sugars are available and consistent with an overall healthy eating plan. Milk and milk products provide nutrients that include calcium and vitamin D[6] (if this vitamin is added by the food manufacturer), vitamin A, potassium, and magnesium. Most people should aim to consume 3 cups of fat-free or low-fat milk or milk products that provide the equivalent amount of calcium each day.

If you don't or can't consume milk, consider ways to supplement your diet with calcium from lactose-free milk products and calcium-fortified foods and beverages. For examples, see appendix B-4, page 332.

Look for the % DV for calcium on the Nutrition Facts label so you know how much 1 serving contributes to the total amount of daily calcium you need. Remember, a food or beverage with 20% DV or more contributes a lot of calcium to your daily total, while one with 5% DV or less contributes a little.

Health experts provide advice about calcium in milligrams (mg), but the Nutrition Facts label lists only a % DV for calcium. Most adults should get

What if I'm lactose-intolerant?

If you want to use milk alternatives because of lactose intolerance, one way to still get the health benefits associated with milk and milk product consumption is to choose alternatives within the milk food group. Try yogurt or lactose-free milk, or take the enzyme lactase before consuming milk products.

What if I avoid milk products?

Choose non-dairy sources of the nutrients provided by milk, including potassium, vitamin A, and magnesium, in addition to calcium and vitamin D. Appendix B can help you make these choices.

---

[6] Older adults, people with dark skin, and people who don't get enough sunlight need more vitamin D. For more information, see chapter 11, "Healthier Older Adults," on page 73 and part V, page 263.

approximately 1,000 mg or 100% DV daily. However, adolescents and teenagers should consume 1,300 mg (130% DV), and post-menopausal women need 1,200 mg (120% DV).

How much milk or milk products do I need?

Look at "My Healthy Eating Plan." How much milk or milk products do you need each day? How does this number sound to you? Does it seem like a lot? Or do you usually eat and drink that much each day?

Let's look at Jennifer's plan:

ABOUT JENNIFER

Jennifer should be eating and drinking 3 cups of fat-free or low-fat milk or equivalent milk products each day based on her calorie needs. She needs to figure out how to spread this out throughout the day. First, she asked herself what milk and milk products and calcium-fortified products she likes. Jennifer wrote down the following:

Favorite milk and milk products: fat-free milk, ice cream, cheese, and yogurt

Favorite calcium-fortified products: orange juice and soy drink

Next, Jennifer thought about which fat-free and low-fat versions of these foods she can eat and how she could plan to eat those foods throughout the day. As we reviewed before, she usually eats lunch with her co-workers and fat-free milk isn't available at the places where they eat. She often drinks a glass of fat-free milk with dinner and has a fat-free yogurt for breakfast. Therefore, she usually needs to get 1 more serving of fat-free or low-fat calcium food in the day. Knowing that, she will add 1 more serving by including a calcium-fortified soy drink as an afternoon snack. She now is set for the day for her calcium-rich foods:

Breakfast: medium banana, *fat-free peach yogurt,* and coffee with *fat-free milk*
Lunch: turkey, with whole wheat roll; romaine lettuce, tomato, and cucumber, with light Italian dressing; medium orange; and unsweetened iced tea
Snack: *calcium-fortified soy drink*
Dinner: pasta and bean salad (1 cup whole wheat pasta, 1/2 cup chickpeas, 1 cup chopped vegetables [carrots, green peppers, and onions], with olive oil) and *1 cup of fat-free milk*
Dessert: raspberries (1 cup)

Now, it's your turn. Write down the milk and milk products you like to drink and eat, in the space below. You should also write sources of non-dairy calcium if this fits your eating style. If you need any ideas, look at the dairy and non-dairy sources of calcium in appendix B, on pages 332 to 333.

Calcium-rich sources I like (milk and milk products or non-dairy sources of calcium):

_____

_____

_____

_____

_____

_____

Now, write down fat-free and low-fat versions of these foods you like or could try and how you could eat and drink those foods and drinks throughout the day.

Breakfast:

_____

Lunch:

_____

Dinner:

_____

Snack:

_____

Dessert:

_____

What to watch for. Unhealthy fats such as saturated and *trans* fats and cholesterol are found in many kinds of milk and milk products. So, look for choices that are fat-free or low-fat when selecting those products. Additionally, some milk products and non-diary desserts and creamers may be

	% DV
Total Fat 12g	**18%**
Saturated Fat 3g	**15%**
Trans Fat 3g	
Cholesterol 30mg	**10%**

processed or made with certain oils (for example, palm oil, palm fruit oil, palm kernel oil, coconut oil, or hydrogenated and partially hydrogenated vegetable oils) that increase the amount of saturated and/or *trans* fats in the food.

The Nutrition Facts label can help you choose fats wisely. Use the % DV on the Nutrition Facts label to identify which nutrients (total fat, saturated fat, and cholesterol) are high or low: 5% DV or less is low and 20% DV or more is high...remember? There is no % DV for *trans* fat, but you should aim to keep *trans* fat as low as possible.

Additionally, the labels on some food packages have information about the specific amount or type of fat in a food. Some examples of claims to look for are "fat-free," "low saturated fat," or "light."

There are many ways to reduce the saturated fat from milk and milk products in your diet. This table shows a few examples of the saturated fat content of different forms of milk and milk products you may eat. Compare foods in the same food category (for example, regular cheddar cheese and low-fat cheddar cheese)—if you choose a lower-saturated fat choice, you can still enjoy many of your favorite foods as you take steps toward a Healthier You.

Food Category	Amount	Saturated Fat Content (grams)	Saturated Fat % Daily Value[a]	Calories
Cheese				
• Regular cheddar cheese	1 oz	6.0	30	114
• Low-fat cheddar cheese	1 oz	1.2	6	49
Milk				
• Whole milk (3.5%)	1 cup	4.6	23	146
• Low-fat (1%) milk	1 cup	1.5	8	102
Frozen desserts				
• Regular ice cream	½ cup	4.9	25	145
• Frozen yogurt, low-fat	½ cup	2.0	10	110

[a] % DVs listed in this column are based on the food amounts listed in the table and on a 2,000-calorie reference diet. The DV for total fat is 65 grams and for saturated fat is 20 grams.

SOUND BITES:

- At the beginning of a meal, ask yourself how much fat-free or low-fat milk and equivalent milk products or other good sources of calcium you've eaten or drunk that day. Then, try to add 1 or 2 servings of these foods if you still haven't met your goals for the day.
- When eating or drinking milk and milk products, look on their Nutrition Facts label to check the calorie and nutrient content and look for those lower in fat, saturated and *trans* fats, cholesterol, and sodium.
- Put milk and milk products on your shopping list for the store. Some milk products vary in their calcium content; therefore, use the % DV to compare products.
- When eating at a restaurant, ask the server whether they serve fat-free or low-fat milk.

Eat whole grains.

Whole grains are an important source of dietary fiber and other nutrients.[7] Healthful diets rich in dietary fiber have been shown to have a number of beneficial effects, including decreasing risk of coronary heart disease and promoting regularity. Some examples of whole-grain products could include whole wheat bread, whole wheat cereal, and brown rice.

But, wait a minute. Have you heard carbohydrates are bad? That we should not be eating them? Well, that's not true. So, we are here to help clear up the issue. Foods containing carbohydrates are an essential part of a healthful diet. In addition to whole grains, healthy foods that provide carbohydrates, as well as many other nutrients, are fruits, vegetables, and fat-free and low-fat milk products. Unfortunately, many of us don't always choose the best carbohydrate foods. There are some foods with carbohydrates with added sugars or added fats we need to watch out for: cakes, cookies, crackers, candy, and doughnuts, to name a few.

Foods with carbohydrates that many of us need to eat more of are those that contain dietary fiber. One example is whole grains. In addition, some refined grains can be good for us because they may be fortified with folic acid and other essential nutrients, which we discussed in chapter 5, "A Calorie Is a Calorie, or Is It?"

---

[7] Fruits and vegetables are also important sources of dietary fiber.

OK, we know we are throwing a lot of terms out there…whole grains, refined grains, and fortified foods. A more detailed explanation is on pages 284 to 285, in part V, but here is a brief explanation: Whole grains are just that—whole. Nothing has been added or taken away by processing. When whole grains are processed, some of the dietary fiber and other important nutrients are removed. A processed grain is called a refined grain. Some refined grain products have key nutrients, such as folic acid and iron, that were removed during the initial processing and added back. These are called enriched grains. White rice and white bread are enriched grain products. If you read the packaging for these foods, you will see the word "enriched." Some enriched grain foods have extra nutrients added. These are called fortified grains. Many ready-to-eat cereals are fortified.

You may be asking yourself, "What is the bottom line?" Here it is: At least half of the grains you eat should be whole-grain; other grains should be fortified or enriched. We have an easy way for you to remember: Make at least half your grains whole.

Whole grains are an important source of fiber. Many packaged foods have fiber information on the front of the package. For example, the package might say "excellent source of fiber," "contains fiber," "rich in fiber," or "high in fiber." The Nutrition Facts label will list the amount of dietary fiber in a serving and the percent Daily Value (% DV). Look at the % DV column—5% DV or less is low in dietary fiber and 20% DV or more is high.

Check the product name and ingredient list. For many but not all "whole-grain" food products, the words "whole" or "whole grain" may appear before the name (for example, whole wheat bread). Remember, though, since whole-grain foods cannot necessarily be identified by their color or name (for example, brown bread, 9-grain bread, hearty grains bread, and mixed grain bread are not always whole-grain), you need to look at the ingredient list. The whole grain should be the first ingredient listed. The following are some examples of how whole grains could be listed:

- whole wheat
- quinoa
- whole oats/oatmeal
- sorghum
- whole-grain corn
- popcorn
- millet

- wild rice
- brown rice
- buckwheat
- whole rye
- bulgur (cracked wheat)
- whole-grain barley
- triticale

How much dietary fiber do you need? The recommended dietary fiber intake is 14 grams (g) per 1,000 calories consumed. Yes, we know—more counting. But take heart—your healthy heart, that is—much of the time, the grams of fiber are already counted for you on the Nutrition Facts label. The more calories you need, the more fiber your body needs. And, that is why the more calories you need, the more servings of fruits, vegetables, and whole grains you get to eat. Ahh…so there really is some logic behind all of this.

tip
how to spot a whole grain:

Check the ingredient list. **The whole grain should be the first ingredient.**

How many servings of grains should I be eating?

Look at "My Healthy Eating Plan." How many servings of grains do you need each day? How does this number sound to you? Does it seem like a lot? Or, do you usually eat that much each day? Do you usually eat too many servings each day?

Let's look at Jennifer's plan on the next page and see how she fit in her grains.

Now, it's your turn. Write down, in the space below, the whole-grain and fortified and enriched grain foods you like to eat.

Whole-grain foods I like are:

_____

_____

Fortified and enriched grain foods I like are:

_____

_____

Now, write down on the next page when you could consume these foods throughout the day.

Breakfast: _____

Lunch: _____

Dinner: _____

Snack: _____

Dessert: _____

ABOUT JENNIFER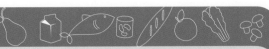

Jennifer should eat 6 to 8 servings of grains each day based on her calorie needs. She figured out how to spread this out throughout the day. First, she asked herself which whole-grain products she likes. She also asked herself what fortified grain products she likes. Jennifer wrote down the following:

Favorite whole-grain products: whole oat squares cereal, whole wheat bread, and whole wheat pasta

Favorite fortified or enriched grain products: many cereals, white rice, French bread, and bagels

Next, Jennifer thought about how she could plan to eat these foods throughout the day. Keeping in mind what we know about Jennifer's eating habits, let's look at what she is planning to eat.

Breakfast: medium banana, fat-free peach yogurt, and coffee with fat-free milk
Lunch: turkey, with *whole wheat roll (3 servings)*; romaine lettuce, tomato, and cucumber, with light Italian dressing; medium orange; and unsweetened iced tea
Snack: calcium-fortified soy drink and *whole oat squares cereal (1 cup = 2 servings)*
Dinner: *pasta and bean salad* ([*1 cup of pasta = 2 servings*], ¹/₂ cup chickpeas, 1 cup chopped vegetables [carrots, green peppers, and onions], with olive oil) and 1 cup of fat-free milk
Dessert: raspberries (1 cup)

Jennifer has enough grains in her diet. She also has at least half of them as whole grains (5 of the 7 servings are whole grains).

Which foods contain dietary fiber and how much do they contain? Here are some examples.

Food	Grams of Fiber	% DV
½ cup navy beans, cooked	9.5	38[a]
½ cup ready-to-eat 100% bran cereal	8.8	35
½ cup lentils, cooked	7.8	31
½ cup chickpeas, cooked	6.2	25
1 medium baked sweet potato, with skin	4.8	19
1 small pear, raw	4.3	17
1 medium baked potato, with skin	3.8	15
½ cup frozen spinach, cooked	3.5	14
1 medium orange, raw	3.1	12
½ cup broccoli, cooked	2.8	11

[a] % DVs listed in this column are based on the food amounts listed in the table and a 2,000-calorie reference diet. The DV for dietary fiber is 25 grams.

Let's do a check on Jennifer's selections for the day to estimate whether she ate enough fiber. Below is a list of Jennifer's food choices and on the next page, an estimate of the grams of fiber in the foods.

ABOUT JENNIFER

Breakfast: *medium banana*, fat-free peach yogurt, and coffee with fat-free milk

Lunch: turkey, with *whole wheat roll (3 servings)*; *romaine lettuce, tomato, and cucumber*, with light Italian dressing; *medium orange*; and unsweetened iced tea

Snack: calcium-fortified soy drink and *whole oat squares cereal (1 cup = 2 servings)*

Dinner: *pasta and bean salad (1 cup pasta, ½ cup chickpeas, 1 cup chopped vegetables [carrots, green peppers, and onions]*, with olive oil) and 1 cup of fat-free milk

Dessert: *raspberries (1 cup)*

Fiber-containing foods on Jennifer's menu:

Banana, medium—3 grams of fiber

Whole wheat roll—6 grams of fiber

Lettuce, tomato, and cucumber (1 cup)—4 grams of fiber

Orange, medium—2 grams of fiber

Whole oat squares cereal—12 grams of fiber

Raspberries—8 grams of fiber

Total estimated fiber = 41 grams

Jennifer's estimated fiber need = 14 g/1,000 calories x 2,000 calories = 28 grams.

She's done a great job at meeting her fiber needs!

Last stop, protein!

You may be thinking to yourself, where's the beef? And you can eat it—if you like beef. Try to select lean cuts such as top round and sirloin. You should also eat poultry, fish, eggs, nuts, seeds, and legumes. Legumes, you may be wondering? You know them, but perhaps by another name—dry beans or peas such as lentils, chickpeas, and kidney beans—see, you do know them!

While meat can be a good source of iron,[8] it isn't best for your body if you eat meat every day because it often contains saturated fat. There are so many protein choices out there—try to vary the ones you eat. Some protein sources are high in fat or prepared in ways that are high in fat, so we need to watch how much we eat and how we prepare them. We'll talk more about fat in the next chapter, so we'll stick to the basics of protein choices here.

How much meat, poultry, fish, eggs, nuts, seeds, and legumes should I be eating?
Look at "My Healthy Eating Plan." How much meat, poultry, fish, eggs, nuts, seeds, and legumes do you need each day? How does this number sound to you? Does it seem like a lot? Or do you usually eat that much each day? Do you usually eat too much each day?

---

[8] Teenage girls and women of childbearing age need additional iron. They can get iron from meat, poultry, and fish, from vegetables such as spinach, and from iron-fortified foods combined with an enhancer of iron absorbtion, such as a vitamin C source (for example, orange juice). For more information, see appendix B-3, page 331, and appendix B-9, page 339.

Let's look at Jennifer's eating plan:

ABOUT JENNIFER

Jennifer should eat 2 or fewer servings of lean meat, poultry, or fish and 1 serving of nuts, seeds, or legumes on most days based on her calorie needs. She figured out how to spread this out throughout the day. First, she asked herself which meat, poultry, and fish she likes. She also asked herself which nuts, seeds, and legumes she likes. Jennifer wrote down the following:

Favorite meat, poultry, and fish: chicken, turkey, salmon, and tuna

Favorite nuts, seeds, and legumes: lentils, peanuts, peanut butter, sunflower seeds, chickpeas, and kidney beans

Next, she thought about how she could plan to eat these foods through-out the day. She is eating approximately 3 oz of turkey at lunch. That's 1 serving of meat, poultry, or fish. She's planning to eat $1/2$ cup of chick-peas at dinner, which is 1 serving of nuts, seeds, and legumes.

Breakfast: medium banana, fat-free peach yogurt, and coffee with fat-free milk
Lunch: *turkey (3 oz = 1 serving)*, with whole wheat roll; romaine lettuce, tomato, and cucumber, with light Italian dressing; medium orange; and unsweetened iced tea
Snack: calcium-fortified soy drink and whole oat squares cereal
Dinner: *pasta and bean salad* (1 cup pasta, $1/2$ *cup chickpeas*, 1 cup chopped vegetables [carrots, green peppers, and onions], with olive oil) and 1 cup of fat-free milk
Dessert: raspberries (1 cup)

Now, it's your turn. Write down the meat, poultry, fish, eggs, nuts, seeds, and legumes you like to eat, on the next page.

Meat, poultry, fish, and eggs I like are:

_____

_____

Nuts, seeds, and legumes I like are:

_____

_____

Now, write down when you could eat these foods throughout the day.

Breakfast:

_____

Lunch:

_____

Dinner:

_____

Snack:

_____

Dessert:

_____

tip
for choosing lean cuts of beef:

Look for cuts that have *loin* or *round* in their name such as sirloin and eye of round.

Congratulations! Now, you have completed one full-day healthy eating plan that is made by you, for you. And guess what? Not only is it healthy, but it is full of foods you already love. You can take the list of foods you have created in each food group and make substitutions in your full-day menu to give yourself more menu options. The more you do this, the easier it will get and the more knowledge you will have. Knowledge is power, and options offer flexibility. You are on your way to a Healthier You.

Part IV of this book gives you recipes and ideas to help you expand your daily choices—when you are ready. We know that it takes time to adjust and refine your diet until you are comfortable. Take it slowly; take it at your own pace. Remember: Small steps lead to big rewards.

In the next chapter, we'll talk more about adjusting the food choices you make to help you gain even more health benefits from the foods you choose. We'll talk more about fat—and making healthy-fat food choices—sound interesting? And we'll talk about sweets and salt. You have learned a lot about food groups and healthy food choices—you should be proud.

Summing it up

Mix up your choices within each food group:

- *Focus on fruits.* Eat a variety of fruits—whether fresh, frozen, canned, or dried—rather than fruit juice, for most of your fruit choices. For a 2,000-calorie diet, you will need 2 cups of fruit each day (for example, 1 small banana, 1 medium orange, and ¼ cup of dried apricots or peaches add up to 2 cups).
- *Vary your veggies.* Eat more dark green veggies such as broccoli, kale, and other dark leafy greens; orange veggies such as carrots, sweet potatoes, pumpkin, and winter squash; and beans and peas such as pinto beans, kidney beans, black beans, garbanzo beans, split peas, and lentils. For a 2,000-calorie diet, you will need 2½ cups of vegetables each day.
- *Get your calcium-rich foods.* Get 3 cups of fat-free or low-fat milk—or an equivalent amount of low-fat yogurt and/or low-fat cheese (1½ ounces of cheese equals 1 cup of milk)—every day. For kids ages 2 to 8, it's 2 cups of milk. If you don't or can't consume milk, choose lactose-free milk products and/or calcium-fortified foods and beverages.
- *Make half your grains whole.* Eat at least 3 ounces of whole-grain cereals, breads, crackers, rice, or pasta every day. One ounce is about 1 slice of bread, 1 cup of breakfast cereal, or ½ cup of cooked rice or pasta. Look to see that grains such as wheat, rice, oats, or corn are referred to as "whole" in the list of ingredients.
- *Go lean with protein.* Choose lean meats and poultry. Bake it, broil it, or grill it and take the skin off poultry. And vary your protein choices—with more fish, dry beans, peas, nuts, and seeds.

Chapter 8. Fats, Added Sugars, and Salt

Moving on from food groups…it's time to talk about how to choose healthy fats within your calorie needs and how to limit unhealthy fats, added sugars, and salt. Let's start with fats. To do this, you'll need "My Healthy Eating Plan." You have two more areas left that you need to fill out: fats and oils, and sweets.

The skinny on fats

Fats and oils are part of a healthy diet and play many important roles in the body. Fat provides energy and is a carrier of important nutrients such as vitamins A, D, E, and K and carotenoids. But fat can impact the health of our hearts and arteries in a positive or negative way, depending on the types of fat we eat. Experts recommend getting between 20 and 35 percent of calories from total fat, with most fats coming from sources of "good" fat, such as fish, nuts, and vegetable oils.

SOUND BITES:

- Eat less saturated and *trans* fats, and cholesterol.
- Be wise about fats by eating fish, nuts, and foods with or prepared with vegetable oils.
- Use the label to choose fats wisely.

Limit saturated and *trans* fats, and cholesterol. Eating too many saturated and *trans* fats, or cholesterol, may raise the level of LDL (bad) cholesterol and increase the risk of heart disease. A saturated fat, the type of fat that is solid at room temperature, is found mostly in animal-based food products. A *trans* fat is made when liquid vegetable oil is processed to become solid. And cholesterol is a fatty substance found only in animal-based products like egg yolks and whole milk. It is important to eat less than 10 percent of your calories from saturated fats. How do we figure this out?

For example, if you aim to eat 2,000 calories per day, your daily allowance of saturated fat would be less than 10 percent of 2,000 calories or 200 calories. There are approximately 9 calories in a gram of fat. OK, OK. To make the math easier, we'll use 10 calories per gram of fat. This at least gives you the right idea. Therefore, 200 calories/10 g/cal. = 20 or 20 grams—which equals 100% DV for saturated fat. This table shows the saturated fat limits for people with various calorie needs. Also, you should keep *trans* fats as low as possible, and eat less than 300 milligrams of cholesterol each day. These limits are recommended so you will not consume too much saturated fat and too many calories in your healthy eating plan.

Total Calorie Intake	Limit of Saturated Fat Intake
1,600	18 g or less
2,000	20 g or less
2,200	24 g or less
2,500	25 g or less
2,800	31 g or less

Unhealthy fats such as saturated and *trans* fats, and cholesterol, are found in many foods. So, look for choices that are lean, fat-free, or low-fat when selecting and preparing meat, poultry, dry beans, and milk products. An easy and quick way to reduce saturated fats is to trim excess fat from meat and poultry and remove the skin from poultry. Additionally, watch out for foods processed or made with certain oils (for example, palm oil, palm fruit oil, palm kernel oil, and coconut oil) that increase the amount of saturated fats in the food. Examples of foods that tend to have saturated fats are fatty cuts of meat, whole milk products, cakes, cookies, pies, crackers, candy, candy bars, household shortening, and creamers. Limiting these foods can reduce saturated fats in your diet.

Trans fats are mostly found in food products made with shortening and partially hydrogenated vegetable oils—liquid oil that is processed to become a solid fat. Most of the *trans* fats Americans eat come from cakes, cookies, crackers, pies, fried potatoes, household shortening, and hard (stick) margarine. Look for partially hydrogenated oil in the ingredient list—and limit these foods. Limiting consumption of many processed foods is a good way to reduce *trans* and saturated fats.

Use the label—what to look for and how it adds up.
Use the % DV on the Nutrition Facts label to identify whether total fat, saturated fat, and cholesterol are high or low. Remember: 5% DV or less is low and 20% DV or more is high. There is no % DV for *trans* fat, but you should aim to keep *trans* fat intake as low as possible.

	% DV
Total Fat 12g	**18%**
Saturated Fat 3g	**15%**
Trans Fat 3g	
Cholesterol 30mg	**10%**

Additionally, the front of many food packages has information called claims that describe a specific level of fat in a food. Some examples of claims to look for are "fat-free," "low saturated fat," or "light."

There are many ways to reduce saturated fats in your diet. The table on the next page shows a few examples of the saturated fat content of different forms of foods you may eat. Compare foods in the same food type (for example, regular cheddar cheese and low-fat cheddar cheese). You can choose the one with less saturated fat and still eat many of the foods you enjoy.

Be wise about fat. Choose fats found in fish, nuts, and vegetable oils. Most of the fat in your diet should come from sources of what are called polyunsaturated and monounsaturated fat. You may have heard of polyunsaturated fats such as omega-6 and omega-3 fatty acids. It's a mouthful, we know, but a mouthful of these fats is good for you in moderation to replace the saturated and *trans* fats you have chosen to cut back on. As we mentioned before, experts recommend getting between 20 and 35 percent of calories from *total* fat, with most fats coming from fish, nuts, and vegetable oils. And we've made it easier for you to get these amounts of fat by following the food group recommendations. Look at the table below, and see whether you can add any foods there to your repertoire of foods in "My Healthy Eating Plan." One more word of caution about fats: calories. Foods that are high in fats are usually high in calories.

Monounsaturated Fatty Acids	Polyunsaturated Omega-6 Fatty Acids	Polyunsaturated Omega-3 Fatty Acids
Nuts	Vegetable oils:	Walnuts
Vegetable oils:	Soybean	Flaxseed
Canola	Corn	Certain fish[a]:
Olive	Safflower	Salmon
High oleic safflower		Trout
Sunflower		Herring
		Vegetable oils:
		Soybean
		Canola

[a] Women who may become pregnant, pregnant women, nursing mothers, and young children should avoid some types of fish and eat types lower in mercury. See www.cfsan.fda.gov/~dms/admehg3.html or call 1-888-SAFEFOOD for more information.

Food Category[a]	Portion	Saturated Fat Content (grams)	Saturated Fat % Daily Value[b]	Calories
Cheese				
• Regular cheddar cheese	1 oz	6.0	30	114
• Low-fat cheddar cheese	1 oz	1.2	6	49
Ground beef				
• Regular ground beef (25% fat)	3 oz (cooked)	6.1	31	236
• Extra lean ground beef (5% fat)	3 oz (cooked)	2.6	13	148
Milk				
• Whole milk (3.25%)	1 cup	4.6	23	146
• Low-fat (1%) milk	1 cup	1.5	8	102
Breads				
• Croissant (med)	1 medium	6.6	33	231
• Bagel, oat bran (4")	1 medium	0.2	1	227
Frozen desserts				
• Regular ice cream	1/2 cup	4.9	25	145
• Frozen yogurt, low-fat	1/2 cup	2.0	10	110
Table spreads				
• Butter	1 tsp	2.4	12	34
• Soft margarine with zero *trans* fats	1 tsp	0.7	4	25
Chicken				
• Fried chicken (leg with skin)	3 oz (cooked)	3.3	17	212
• Roasted chicken (breast, no skin)	3 oz (cooked)	0.9	5	140
Fish				
• Fried fish	3 oz	2.8	14	195
• Baked fish	3 oz	1.5	8	129

[a] Source: Agricultural Research Service (ARS) Nutrient Database for Standard Reference, Release 17.

[b] % DVs listed in this column are based on the food amounts listed in the table.

Added sugars

We talked about added sugars in the last chapter when discussing carbohydrates. You also may have noticed that in "My Healthy Eating Plan," there is a place for you to add sweets. Sweets could include foods that have added sugars like ice cream, cookies, some breakfast cereals, fruit drinks, and fruit yogurt. This might seem tricky when you look on a Nutrition Facts label. The only information you will see there is the total amount of sugar (added sugar and naturally occurring sugars) in a food. That's OK. We are going to help make this information clearer. Let's get started.

The Nutrition Facts label lists how many grams of sugar the food contains, but does not list added sugars separately. The amount listed includes sugars that are naturally present in foods (such as the fructose and sucrose in fruit, or the lactose in milk) and sugars added to the food during processing or preparation.

Added sugars, also known as caloric sweeteners, provide calories but few or no vitamins and minerals. So, the more foods with added sugars you eat, the more difficult it can be to get the nutrients you require within your calorie needs. And, if you go over your calorie needs, you may gain weight. Our goal is to choose and prepare foods and beverages with *little* added sugars.

How do you know whether a food contains added sugars? On packaged foods, look on the ingredient list. The ingredients are listed in order of amount by weight from most to least. Foods that have added sugars as one of the first few ingredients may be high in total sugars. Check the Nutrition Facts label to determine the amount of sugars per serving of the food. The sugars listed include naturally occurring sugars (like those in fruit and milk) as well as those added to a food or drink. When you see sugar on the Nutrition Facts label, you can visualize the total amount of sugar (natural and added) in 1 serving of a food item: 4 grams of sugar = ~1 teaspoon = ~16 calories. For example, a 12-fluid ounce soft drink with 150 calories typically has almost the equivalent of 10 teaspoons of sugar.

Names for added sugars in an ingredient list include brown sugar, corn sweetener, corn syrup, dextrose, fructose, fruit juice concentrates, glucose, high fructose corn syrup, honey, invert sugar, lactose, maltose, malt syrup, molasses, raw sugar, sucrose, and syrup. On the next page is an example of an ingredient list of a fruit yogurt, and the added sugar is circled. Also, check the front of the food package for guidance. Sometimes, the label will say "sugar-free" or "no added sugars."

INGREDIENTS: Cultured Grade A reduced fat milk, apples, high fructose corn syrup, cinnamon, nutmeg, natural flavors, and pectin. Contains active yogurt and *L. acidophilus* cultures.

Foods from restaurants, convenience stores, or other food stores may also have added sugar. The foods that contribute the most added sugars to diets of Americans are regular soft drinks; sugar and candy; cakes, cookies, and pies; fruit drinks such as fruit punch; sweetened milk and milk products such as ice cream, sweetened yogurt, and sweetened milk; and sweetened grains such as sugar-sweetened cereals, cinnamon toast, and honey-nut waffles. We hope the sugar story is getting clearer.

Now, you may be looking at "My Healthy Eating Plan" and wondering, "How does this all go to-gether?" You may think that there are not many options for sweets in a healthy eating plan. Well, unfortunately, this is true in one sense. There isn't a lot of room in a healthy eating plan for cakes, cookies, pies, regular soft drinks, and other sugar-loaded foods without gaining weight. It's that simple. But there are ways that we can make a little more room in the healthy eating plan to allow for those foods, occasionally. We will discuss that in chapter 9, "The Balancing Act: Food and Physical Activity." But first, let's get to our last topic in this chapter: Salt.

Sad but true: Chocolate is not a food group!

Salt

Nearly all of us eat too much salt (sodium). On average, the more salt a person eats, the higher his or her blood pressure is. Most salt we eat comes from processed foods, not necessarily from the salt shaker. Some people are surprised by this, and that is why we are going to talk about the Nutrition Facts label again—you'll see "salt" listed as sodium there. For our purposes, we can use the terms "salt" and "sodium" interchangeably.

Some people should get no more than 1,500 milligrams of sodium each day, and should meet the potassium recommendation through foods. These people are:

- individuals with high blood pressure
- African-Americans/ blacks
- middle-aged or older adults.

Consult your health care provider for advice on how much sodium and potassium you should get.

Eating less salt is an important way to reduce the risk of high blood pressure, which may in turn reduce the risk of heart disease, stroke, congestive heart failure, and kidney damage.

In addition to eating less salt, other lifestyle changes may prevent or delay getting high blood pressure and may help lower high blood pressure. These lifestyle changes include eating more potassium-rich foods, losing excess weight, being more physically active, and eating a healthy diet. Let's see, we talked briefly about potassium in chapter 5, "A Calorie Is a Calorie, or Is It?" We'll mention it again here to emphasize the importance of eating potassium-rich foods.

tips
for eating less salt:

- When you're choosing packaged foods, look at the sodium content on the Nutrition Facts label. Use the percent Daily Value (% DV) to help limit your sodium intake. 5% DV or less is low and 20% DV or more is high. You don't want to exceed a total of 100% DV for sodium in a day. Some people (people with high blood pressure, African-Americans/blacks, and people who are middle-aged or older) should get even less—about half as much.

- Compare sodium content for similar foods. This can really make a difference. The table on the next page shows you examples of foods that have a range of sodium content depending on the brand chosen. By comparing brands of similar foods, you can save over hundreds of milligrams of sodium. Use the Nutrition Facts label on the food package to select food brands that are lower in sodium.

- Use the claims on the front of the food package to quickly identify foods that contain less salt or that are a good source of potassium, a nutrient you want to get more of in your daily diet. Examples include "low in sodium," "very low sodium," and "high in potassium."

- When you're preparing food at home, use herbs and spices to add flavor to your foods so you don't depend too heavily on salt. Don't salt foods before or during cooking—and limit salt use at the table.

- When you're eating out, ask that your meal be prepared without added salt or ask the server to identify foods on the menu that are made without added salt.

OK…so nearly all of us eat too much salt, and most of us don't get enough potassium—it is no wonder so many of us have high blood pressure! Here's what you need to know about sodium and potassium.

Everyone should get no more than 2,300 milligrams of sodium each day. People with high blood pressure, African-Americans/blacks, and people who are middle-aged or older should get even less, because sodium from salt can affect those folks more than others.

As you decrease the amount of salt you eat, your taste for salt will gradually decrease—and *you won't miss it.* Adding spices to foods makes them more flavorful—another way to help you decrease the amount of salt you use when cooking. We've provided a tip sheet in part IV, "Recipes and Resources," for ways to use spices instead of salt when preparing food.

The table below shows the importance of reading the food label to determine the sodium content of food. The sodium content, shown below in milligrams, or mg, can often differ significantly between similar foods or brands.

Food Group	Amount	Range of Sodium Content (mg)	% Daily Value (% DV)[a] for Sodium
Breads, all types	1 oz	95–210	4–9
Frozen pizza, plain, cheese	4 oz	450–1,200	19–50
Frozen vegetables, all types	½ cup	2–160	0–7
Salad dressing, regular fat, all types	2 Tbsp	110–505	5–21
Salsa	2 Tbsp	150–240	6–10
Soup (tomato), reconstituted	8 oz	700–1,260	29–53
Tomato juice	8 oz (~1 cup)	340–1,040	14–43
Potato chips[b]	1 oz (28.4 g)	120–180	5–8
Tortilla chips[b]	1 oz (28.4 g)	105–160	4–7
Pretzels[b]	1 oz (28.4 g)	290–560	12–23

[a] % DVs listed in this column are based on the food amounts listed in the table. The DV for sodium is 2,400 milligrams.

[b] All snack foods are regular flavor, salted.

Source: Agricultural Research Service (ARS) Nutrient Database for Standard Reference, Release 17, and recent manufacturers' label data from retail market surveys. Serving sizes were standardized to be comparable among brands within a food. Pizza and bread slices vary in size and weight across brands.

Note: None of the foods in the ARS Nutrient Database or market surveys were labeled low-sodium products.

Get 4,700 milligrams of potassium each day. You can use the foods listed in appendix B-1, page 328, to add to "My Healthy Eating Plan," to help increase the amount of naturally rich (not fortified) potassium you are getting in your diet. Potassium-containing food sources include leafy greens such as spinach and collards, bananas and fruit from vines such as grapes and blackberries, root vegetables such as carrots and potatoes, and citrus fruits such as oranges and grapefruit.

When buying packaged food, check the Nutrition Facts label to see potassium content. Use the % DV to look for foods that are low in sodium and high in potassium. We do need to warn you that sometimes, potassium is not found on the label—but you've got a good list in appendix B.

Summing it up

Let's sum up what we've learned in this chapter…
- Choose fats found in fish, nuts, and vegetables.
- Know your limits on fats, salt, and sugars.
- Use the Nutrition Facts label on foods. Look for foods low in saturated and *trans* fats, cholesterol, and sodium.
- Choose and prepare foods and beverages with little salt (sodium) and/or added sugars (caloric sweeteners).

Chapter 9. The Balancing Act: Food and Physical Activity

Staying at—or getting to—a healthy weight helps us in several ways. Remember: Not only does it help us get to that "better me," but research shows it plays an important role in reducing the risk of several types of chronic diseases. In chapter 4, "Where to Start," you identified what your healthy weight range is and wrote it down in "My Personal Profile." This chapter will focus on finding the balance between food and physical activity and reaching or maintaining a healthy weight.

If you are overweight or obese, you are not alone. Many of us are. In fact, in the United States, two-thirds of adults are overweight or obese. That is why many of us need to eat fewer calories, be more physically active, and make wiser food choices. What we are going to do in this chapter is sum up the information you have already learned so you can see where you can take small steps to decrease the number of calories you consume if you need to lose weight. We are going to introduce physical activity to you as part of the "energy balance" equation. You will learn more about that in the next chapter.

Losing weight, gaining life

Lifestyle changes in diet and physical activity are the healthiest choices for weight loss. To lose weight, many of us need a reduction in 500 calories or more per day from food and drink. In addition, increasing physical activity is also important. Remember: To lose weight, calories in must be less than calories out.

> **tip**
>
> **Prevent gradual weight gain!**
>
> For most adults, cutting back 50 to 100 calories per day may prevent the gradual weight gain that comes as we get older.

When it comes to weight control, it is calories that count—not the proportions of fat, carbohydrates, and protein in the diet. Diets that provide very low or very high amounts of protein, carbohydrates, or fat are likely not providing enough of some nutrients—that is why they are not advisable for long-term use. Although these kinds of weight-loss diets have been shown to result in weight loss, maintaining weight loss ultimately depends on a change in your lifestyle. A healthy lifestyle is about more than just your weight—it is also about feeling better and reducing your risk of chronic diseases.

"Energy balance"

To maintain your body weight, the energy that you expend through your daily activities (for example, breathing, sleeping, and moving around) and additional physical activities has to equal the energy (food and drink) that you consume as calories. If these two things—energy use and energy consumption—are equal, then you are in "energy balance." If you want to lose weight, you will have to either increase the amount of energy expended through additional physical activities or decrease the calories that you consume, or both. Be careful to still get all the nutrients that you need if you decide to eat fewer calories to tip the energy balance. You will get these important vitamins and minerals if you follow the food group recommendations in "My Healthy Eating Plan." The recommendations provide the right proportions of fat, carbohydrates, and protein for good health. Remember: It is always important to eat foods that are high in nutrients for the number of calories they contain, such as fruits, vegetables, whole grains, and fat-free or low-fat milk or equivalent milk products.

We know it's difficult to lose weight; it is better not to gain it in the first place. Since many of us tend to gain weight slowly as we age, small decreases in calorie intake can help avoid that slow weight gain, especially when accompanied by increased physical activity. Remember: 3,500 calories equals 1 pound. For most adults, a reduction of 50 to 100 calories per day from foods and beverages may prevent gradual weight gain.

Calorie-lowering strategies

The healthiest way to reduce calorie intake is to reduce intake of added sugars, saturated and *trans* fats, and alcohol, which all provide calories but few or no "good for you" nutrients. You already know about added sugars and unhealthy fats. You learned about them in chapters 7 and 8. Let's spend some time discussing alcohol—because it can be a simple way to cut calories out of your diet.

Alcoholic beverages supply calories but few essential nutrients. The next page has a table to help you estimate the calories from various alcoholic beverages. Calories are provided for serving volume of beer, wine, and distilled spirits. Higher alcohol content (higher percent alcohol or higher proof), and mixing alcohol with other beverages, such as sugar-sweetened soft drinks or tonic water, fruit juice, or cream, increases the number of calories in the beverage. You can find information on the health effects of consuming alcohol on page 309, in part V.

As you can see from the table below, each drink has about 100 calories. Remember: You need to reduce your food and drink intake by 3,500 calories or burn 3,500 calories without increasing food intake to lose a pound. If you have one light beer each day, that is 100 extra calories! A cocktail made with a sugar-sweetened mixer could be twice that number of calories or more!

Beverage	Approximate Calories (per 1 fluid oz)	Example Serving Volume	Approximate Total Calories
Beer (regular)	12	12 oz	144
Beer (light)	9	12 oz	108
White wine	20	5 oz	100
Red wine	21	5 oz	105
Sweet dessert wine	47	3 oz	141
80-proof distilled spirits (gin, rum, vodka, and whiskey)	64	1.5 oz	96

The same goes for those of us who drink sugar-sweetened beverages without any alcohol. Many of them have at least 150 calories in 1 serving—usually one 12-fluid ounce can. But often, these beverages come in larger bottles, and we drink the entire bottle—easily 300 to 500 unnecessary calories. If you have one 20-ounce sugar-sweetened beverage each day, in 2 weeks, it can add up to over 3,500 excess calories—or a weight gain of 1 pound.

Another way to reduce calorie intake is to eat foods that are low in calories for the amount of food eaten. Examples of these foods are many kinds of vegetables and fruits and some soups. If a soup is made with cream, it will not count toward this strategy (SORRY), but to double the impact, a soup made with low-sodium broth and packed with vegetables can be low in calories, packed with nutrients, and filling too! Just watch out for the salt content. Remember: It is always important to eat foods that are high in nutrients for the number of calories they contain, such as fruits, vegetables, whole grains, and fat-free or low-fat milk or equivalent milk products.

One more way to reduce calorie intake is to evaluate the portion size of foods. We already know, portion size is the amount of food eaten at one sitting—and, in general, portion size has increased significantly over the past two decades.

For example, the muffin you ate at work 5 years ago may have had 300 calories, but today's muffins are typically larger and may contain up to 500 calories. You may have not noticed the increase—but it could be 200 extra calories! And, science shows us that controlling portion size helps limit calorie intake, particularly when eating calorie-dense foods (foods that are high in calories for a given measure of food). Therefore, it is essential that we understand how portion size—the amount you eat—compares to a recommended standard amount of food (that is, a serving) from each food group at a specific calorie level. Understanding serving size and portion size is important in following "My Healthy Eating Plan." When using packaged foods with a Nutrition Facts label, pay attention to the serving sizes and how they compare to the food amounts in the DASH Eating Plan and USDA Food Guide (in appendix A); you will be surprised!

SOUND BITES:

READ FOOD PACKAGES TO MAKE SMART FOOD CHOICES.

Use the Nutrition Facts label. Most packaged foods have a Nutrition Facts label. Use this tool to make smart food choices and to find information about the amount of calories and nutrients you are eating.

Know your portion size. Controlling portion size helps limit calorie intake, particularly when eating foods that are high in calories. When you eat packaged foods, use the Nutrition Facts label to check servings and calories as noted above. When eating whole foods or packaged foods without labels, pay attention to how the portion size compares to a recommended amount of food from each food group.

Read the ingredient list. Ingredients are listed in order by weight from most to least. Make sure those ingredients you want more of, such as whole grains (for example, whole wheat), are listed first. Make sure ingredients you want to eat less of, like added sugars, are not one of the first few ingredients. Remember: Some names for added sugars (caloric sweeteners) include: sucrose, high fructose corn syrup, corn syrup, corn sweetener, maple syrup, honey, and molasses.

Check for claims on the front of food packages. The labels of some food products have a variety of claims that you can use to help manage your weight such as "low calorie," "lite," "low fat," "reduced fat," or "reduced sugar."

Write it down.

One technique that is useful in looking for ways to cut calories from foods is to write down what we eat. Do it for 1 day. This means writing down everything you eat, along with an estimate of the amount you eat—this time be realistic. If you put a pat of butter on your toast, write down both the toast and a teaspoon of butter—that is, if your pat was a teaspoon! How do you know how much of a food you are eating? Take a minute to look in your cabinet. Find your measuring spoons and cups. Next, find something familiar that you can use to eyeball measurements that you will remember.

tip

For some of us, our thumbprint is about the size of a teaspoon; for others, our thumbprint is about the size of a tablespoon. Try it and see! Another example is our fist. For some of us, our fist is about the size of a 1/2 cup, and for others, it is 1 cup. It doesn't need to be exact, this is just an estimate—and it will help you estimate how much food you are eating.

In part III, "Making a Healthier You Happen," we have included worksheets for you to write down the food you eat in 1 day, for a couple of days. Once you do this, you can look at those foods and find ways that work for you to cut 100 calories here and 100 calories there. Some of the tips we have provided can work for you, but you can also come up with more ways. For example, could you leave the jelly or butter off your morning toast? Use less salad dressing? Avoid high-calorie sauces at dinner-time? Maybe these aren't things that you do every time you eat a food. Do what works for you, but be realistic. A realistic rate of weight loss is 1/2 to 2 pounds per week.

Be more active.

Eating fewer calories, of course, is just one side of the equation. Calorie output needs to be in balance with calorie intake to maintain body weight. That means the calories "burned" during physical activity (in addition to activities of daily living) need to be the same as the calories taken in as food. Here are a few recommendations about how much physical activity we should be doing and how "hard" we should be performing. Don't worry if there are confusing terms; we'll get into the details in the next chapter. But since we have been talking energy balance, we can't wrap up the discussion without talking about physical activity a little bit. So, here we go! For health purposes, all adults should engage in at least 30 minutes of moderate-intensity physical activity on most days of the week. This recommended amount of activity is in addition to light-intensity routine activities of daily living and physical activity of less than 10 minutes. However, to prevent weight gain, adults may need up to 60 minutes of moderate- to vigorous-intensity activity on most days of the week while at the same time not eating more calories than required. To sustain weight loss, adults may need as much as 60 to 90 minutes of moderately intense physical activity per day while not eating too much. More about this in the next chapter....

Chapter 10. Making Physical Activity Part of a Healthier You

Most of us know we need to be physically active to be healthy. It's not new information, but it leaves us with many questions and many opinions. There's plenty of information about physical activity, but sorting through it and figuring out what to do can be challenging. Instead of answering questions, all that information only seems to generate more: "What exactly does being physically active mean? Is this physical activity or 'exercise?' How much do we need versus what can we do to get by? Do we need to do it all at once? Is there an easy way to fit it into our day, because life is pretty hectic already?" So many questions…plus, almost every day, a new exercise product is introduced promising a quick fix—to whip us into shape requiring only the slightest amount of effort on our part. If only that were true, we tell ourselves….

START OFF SMALL
by Lynn Swann*

I have a friend who wanted and needed to lose weight. He went to a trainer and said he wanted to start a workout program. My friend is about 5'4". His weight was north of 300 pounds. The trainer told him to get dressed and walk for as long and as far as he could. After about 20 minutes of walking, he came back and asked the trainer what was next. The trainer said, "That's it. Come back tomorrow." My friend came back the next day and repeated the same 20-minute walk. He continued to walk each day until he could run.... To date, my friend has now run 19 marathons around the world and weighs 165 pounds.

The point: if you just take that first step and consistently stick with it, you can reach high goals. Starting off slowly with small achievable goals and sound advice will ensure safety in your training routine and deter you from giving up. This way you will not be overwhelmed by a large, daunting long-term goal, and you'll gain all the benefits of regular physical activity.

*NFL Hall of Fame Member and Former Chair of the President's Council on Physical Fitness and Sports

Here's what we can agree on—we'll give it to you straight: The basic, scientifically grounded information on physical activity. Then, we'll begin to figure out how to balance this with your day and your lifestyle.

Earlier, in "My Personal Profile," you determined your starting activity level: Sedentary, Moderately Active, or Active. This was part of determining how physically active you currently are and estimating your daily calorie needs, which are key to setting your goals. Whether you are trying to gain, lose, or maintain your weight, physical activity goes hand in hand with good nutrition and overall health.

The basics

Science tells us that when it comes down to our overall health, adults, regardless of age, need to do two key types of physical activities:

- **Cardio or Aerobic[9]:** At a minimum, do moderately intense cardio activity for at least 30 minutes per day, most days of the week.
  AND
- **Strength Training:** At a minimum, 2 days per week.

We are going to introduce a couple of terms that you may be less familiar with in this context—moderately intense and vigorously intense. By understanding how much effort we need to exert, we can begin to choose what kind of activity fits our available time, life, and needs. Here are some tips and examples to help identify whether physical activity is moderately or vigorously intense.

Cardio—What's Your Intensity?

Moderate: While performing the physical activity, if your heart is beating noticeably faster—it's probably moderately intense: We need to do this level of activity for at least 30 minutes, most days of the week.

Examples include:
- walking briskly (a 15-minute mile)
- light yard work (raking/bagging leaves or using a lawn mower)
- light snow shoveling
- actively playing with children
- biking at a casual pace.

[9] Cardio or aerobic exercise is any type of exercise that increases the work of the heart and lungs.

Vigorous: If you are breathing hard and fast and your heart rate is increased substantially during physical activity, it's probably vigorously intense.

Examples include:

- jogging/running
- swimming laps
- rollerblading/inline skating at a brisk pace
- cross-country skiing
- most competitive sports (football, basketball, or soccer)
- jumping rope.

You don't have to do 30 minutes all at once…

To meet the goal of 30 minutes a day of moderately intense physical activity, you don't have to do all 30 minutes at once. Scientific evidence shows you get the same health benefits from breaking 30 minutes up into three 10-minute or two 15-minute intervals throughout the day, if you prefer. Daily activities like climbing several flights of stairs or parking farther away from store entrances are a good start. But if you don't do that activity for at least 10 minutes at a time, it doesn't help you meet the recommendation for 30 minutes of moderately intense physical activity. In addition, for most people, greater health benefits can be obtained by engaging in physical activity of more vigorous intensity or of longer duration.

What is strength training and why do it?

Moving on to the second type of physical activity—strength training. This consists of resistance exercises, which means your muscles work or hold against an applied force or weight. These exercises increase the strength of our muscles, help maintain the integrity of our bones, and may improve our balance, coordination, and mobility. Strength training can also change the appearance of our bodies with better muscle definition. Usually, resistance exercises are done using weights or workout bands, but there are other ways to achieve the same effect. If you like going to the gym, include resistance exercises in your routine there; or look at the examples on the next page and do them at home. Strength training or resistance exercises can be done anywhere. An example of a goal to work toward could be to do 8 to 12 repetitions of 6 to 8 strength-training exercises twice a week.

Examples include:

- push-ups
- pull-ups
- biceps curls
- sit-ups
- carrying full laundry baskets
- rowing a boat
- strength training in aerobics class.

Both strength training and cardio activity are important. In particular, strength training helps develop and maintain healthy bones, and develop and tone muscles.

What's in it for me?

Part of it comes down to: Feeling better! Looking better! Not so bad, right? In the big picture, it also comes down to good physical health. If that's not enough, there's also that sense of well-being you get from regular physical activity—a constructive way to deal with the demands of the day, release stress, and just feel better about yourself. Many people say that exercising regularly helps them have more energy, sleep better, and simply, enjoy taking time to do something good for themselves.

With most everything, extra work really does pay off! Physical activity is no exception, and the more active you are, the more you benefit. For example, you can further reduce your risk for many chronic diseases, including cardiovascular disease, type 2 diabetes, colon and breast cancers, and osteoporosis, by doing more than the minimum 30 minutes of moderate-intensity physical activity on most days of the week. Incorporating up to 60 minutes of cardio activity may also help you to prevent unhealthy weight gain or to manage your weight, if that is your goal.

> "I feel my day isn't complete without some physical activity. I know I miss it on the days I don't do it."
>
> — Eric, age 42

Some of us suffer from the yo-yo factor—weight on, weight off, weight on, weight off. Sure, we can lose the weight, but how do we keep it off for good? That may take at least 60 to 90 minutes of daily moderate-intensity physical activity. Sounds like a lot—no kidding! But it's the truth based on the data of people who have successfully lost weight (at least 30 pounds) and kept it off for at least a year. Keep your perspective and start small—do your physical activity in 10-minute moderately intense increments and build up. Eventually, you will become your own success story.

Different intensities and types of exercise offer different benefits. Cardio or aerobic activities exercise your heart and increase your ability to be physically active for a longer period of time. This type of endurance makes it easier to carry out harder tasks for longer periods of time—whether it's keeping up with your kids or grandchildren, or playing basketball with your co-workers. Strength training or resistance exercises also contribute to muscular endurance. Strength training is especially beneficial as we get older. As we age, we tend to lose bone and muscle mass, making it difficult to carry out everyday activities: getting in and out of a chair, carrying groceries or laundry, or just walking. Together, cardio and strength training work your whole body. Vigorous physical activity (for example, jogging or other aerobic exercises) provides greater health benefits for physical fitness than does moderate physical activity and burns more calories per unit of time. Aside from all the health benefits, what a bonus that it also seems to make us feel better about ourselves.

Now to the biggest challenge: How do we fit this into our life? Our busy, already-pressed-for-time, on-a-budget life? A lot of people have shared their thoughts with us. Here's some of their feedback on what works.

Buddy System: Some days it's hard to talk yourself into an activity. Working with others who are going through the same thing can be motivating, especially when you promised that you would meet for a walk in the park, or a tennis match, or signed up to take a yoga class together. You don't want to let your buddy down. In the process, you end up not letting yourself down either. Buddies can be co-workers, spouses, neighbors, or even faraway friends that you stay in touch with via e-mail and provide encouragement. Heck, your walking buddy can even be your pet!

The Great Outdoors: Opportunities for physical activity may be closer than you think. Take advantage of public parks and pools. There are millions of acres to explore—walk, hike, swim, kayak, canoe, and bike. Also consider being a volunteer. Whether it's leading a hike or cleaning a trail or playground, you are making a difference in your life and others'.

Enjoy What You Do: If aerobicizing in a room full of people isn't your thing, why do it? There are hundreds of activities to choose from. Find something you like and chances are you will stick with it. Maybe you were a swimmer when you were younger, but haven't thought of it since high school. Many local park and recreation facilities, or area schools, have open or lap swims. Some people enjoy walking around a nearby school track, or if you prefer indoors, walk at your local mall. What about hiking at a local, state, or national park; playing in a soccer, volleyball, or softball league; or taking a yoga, Pilates, or tai-chi class a couple days a week? Don't limit yourself. Don't get discouraged. Pick a few activities to try out, rotate them, and slowly you will figure out what works best for you. Trying something new can be fun and give you more confidence to pursue other activities.

At this point, turn to part III, "My Physical Activity Tracker," on page 113. You can tear it out and make copies for your circle of family and friends. Take a look at the physical activity log—and use it to start tracking your progress. If you prefer, you can track it online at www.presidentschallenge.org.

Hmm…before we wrap up this chapter, we think there might be some of you that still need more nudging—the self-professed couch potatoes. The "I don't exercise, don't want to exercise, hate the thought of exercise, 'run' away from exercise" types. Is that you? We are not giving up on you. We are good to go…armed with over 100 ways for those of you who are allergic to exercise to take that first step. Check out www.smallstep.gov, for small steps to increase your physical activity…gradually build up some endurance to keep going…and begin that lifestyle makeover.

Best of all, no matter what your age, physical ability or limitations, or physical activity level, it's never too late to start! Some form of physical activity is right for everyone.

Summing it up

Let's summarize what we've learned about making physical activity part of a Healthier You:

- Be physically active for at least 30 minutes per day, most days of the week.
- All adults, regardless of age, need both cardio or aerobic, and strength training, for overall health.
- Cardio or Aerobic Activities: At a minimum, do at least 30 minutes of cardio or aerobic moderately intense activities (which can be performed in 10-minute intervals), most days of the week.
- Strength Training: Recommended at least 2 days per week. A goal, for example, might be 8 to 12 repetitions of 6 to 8 strength-training exercises.
- Increasing the intensity or the amount of time that you are physically active can have greater health benefits and may be needed to control body weight. About 60 minutes a day may be needed to prevent weight gain.
- At least 60 to 90 minutes of physical activity most days may be needed to prevent regaining weight for the formerly overweight or obese.

Chapter 11. Healthier Older Adults

If you're an older adult or perhaps playing a vital role in taking care of aging parents or grandparents, there are some nutrition and physical activity considerations to keep in mind. Getting older doesn't mean that our quality of life or desire to be our best is any different. In fact, we usually become more aware of our health as we age. Healthful habits can help older adults enjoy daily activities, stay mobile, and be independent. Anytime is a good time to start healthy habits, no matter how old we are.

> "I walk, garden, and do housework. Exercise keeps me limber. Most people don't think I'm my age."
>
> — Vivian, age 78

So, if you are a little older…you can still be healthier. Eating a balanced diet of nutrient-packed foods applies to all of us, but for older adults, a healthy eating plan may require a little more planning. If you have health problems or take medication regularly, it may be important to check with your health care provider for advice about changing your diet or physical activity level.

Fiber, more important than ever

We've talked about how a healthy diet includes fiber-rich foods, such as fruits, vegetables, and whole grains, that offer many health benefits including protection against heart disease. Another benefit is that fiber promotes regularity. Constipation may affect older adults for many reasons—from taking certain medications to drinking less fluid.

How much fiber do you need? The recommended dietary fiber intake is 14 grams per 1,000 calories consumed. So, the more calories you eat, the more fiber your body needs. Now, figure out your fiber needs from your estimated calorie needs in your Personal Profile.

Good sources of dietary fiber include: cooked dry beans and ready-to-eat bran cereal or shredded wheat; pears and berries; dried prunes, figs, and dates; and cooked green peas, Brussels sprouts, sweet potatoes, and spinach (see appendix B-8, on page 337). For a 2,000-calorie diet, you will need 2 1/2 cups of vegetables (a source of fiber and other nutrients) each day. Consuming at least 3 or more ounces of whole grains can reduce the risk of several chronic diseases and may help with weight maintenance.

Fats and your heart

Many of us, especially if we are older, have been told to eat less fat. Fat can impact the health of our heart and arteries in positive and negative ways, depending on the type of fat. All the more reason to stay away from saturated fats, *trans* fats, and cholesterol. Eating too much saturated and *trans* fats, the type of fats that are solid at room temperature, may increase the risk of heart disease. Saturated fats can be found in animal-based products such as milk and milk products, butter, meat, and poultry. And eating too much cholesterol, a fatty substance found only in animal-based products, may also increase the risk of heart disease. It's important to eat less than 10 percent of your calories from saturated fats.

For example, if you aim to eat 2,000 calories per day, your daily allowance of saturated fat would be less than 200 calories or 20 grams—which equals 100% Daily Value (DV) for saturated fat. And, remember, this is a limit, not a goal, meaning you do not need to achieve your DV for saturated fat! Furthermore, you should keep *trans* fats (often found in cakes, cookies, crackers, pies, and breads) as low as possible, and eat less than 300 milligrams per day (mg/day) of cholesterol.

Older adults should pay special attention to certain nutrient needs. For example:

- *Many people over 50 years old* have reduced absorption of vitamin B_{12}. Therefore, they should consume vitamin B_{12} from fortified foods or a dietary supplement.[10]
- *Older adults* tend to need more vitamin D to help maintain bone health. Drinking vitamin D-fortified fat-free or low-fat milk, or fortified orange juice, is a good way to get your vitamin D.[11]
- Since constipation may affect up to 20 percent of people over age 65, older adults should consume foods rich in dietary fiber and drink plenty of water.
- Lifestyle changes can prevent or delay the onset of high blood pressure and can lower elevated blood pressure. These changes include increasing potassium intake, reducing salt intake, eating an overall healthful diet, engaging in regular physical activity, and achieving a healthy weight.

Maybe you are someone who has an elevated LDL (bad) cholesterol level. Definitely, you should follow your health care provider's advice. Those of us with elevated cholesterol may be advised to decrease our calories from saturated fat to less than 7 percent of total calories—which is about 16 grams or about 80% DV—and less than 200 mg/day of cholesterol. It's critical to find out what's right for a Healthier You.

[10] Older adults should meet their vitamin B_{12} needs by eating foods fortified with vitamin B_{12}, such as fortified cereals, or by taking the crystalline form of vitamin B_{12} in supplements.

[11] For example, an older adult could get adequate daily vitamin D from 3 cups of milk (300 IU), 1 cup of vitamin D-fortified orange juice (100 IU), plus 600 IU from vitamin D supplements.

Now, a few words about making wise fat choices: an immediate change you can make is to eat monounsaturated and polyunsaturated fats found in fish, nuts, and vegetable oils to reduce saturated fat calories in your diet. In fact, to help reduce the risk of heart disease, some evidence suggests eating approximately 2 servings of fish per week (a total of about 8 ounces) for people who have already had a heart attack. It may reduce their risk of death from cardiovascular disease. For more information on fats and using the Nutrition Facts label to help choose them wisely, turn to chapter 8, "Fats, Added Sugars, and Salt," on page 51.

The relationship between sodium and potassium

Nearly all of us eat too much salt (sodium). As a matter of fact, on average, the more salt we eat, the higher our blood pressure—and most of the salt we eat comes from processed foods, not necessarily from the salt shaker. Surprised? Eating less salt is an important way to reduce the risk of high blood pressure, which may in turn reduce the risk of heart disease, stroke, congestive heart failure, and kidney damage.

Other lifestyle changes may prevent or delay getting high blood pressure. These include eating more foods rich in potassium, losing excess weight, being more physically active, and eating an overall healthy diet.

A diet rich in potassium helps to counterbalance some of sodium's harmful effects on blood pressure. You may need to consult your health care provider for advice on how much sodium and potassium you should get, but in general, older adults should aim to consume no more than 1,500 mg/day (about 60% DV on the food label) of sodium, and meet the potassium recommendation of (4,700 mg/day) by eating potassium-rich food. When choosing packaged foods, check the sodium content on the Nutrition Facts label. Use the percent Daily Value (% DV) discussed in chapter 8, "Fats, Added Sugars, and Salt," to help limit your sodium intake. Older adults should not exceed about 60% DV for sodium for the day.

Keeping your food safe

Did you know that, every year, an estimated 76 million people in the United States become ill from food that contains harmful bacteria? Older adults are at higher risk. Perhaps, foodborne illness has affected you, and you did not even recognize the common symptoms—an upset stomach, diarrhea, a fever, vomiting, abdominal cramps, and dehydration. It can also result in more severe illness, such as paralysis and meningitis, or even death.

It's important that older adults, people with weakened immune systems, and individuals with certain chronic illnesses pay extra attention and carefully follow food safety advice. Here are simple steps that you and your family can take to minimize the risk—four key words: clean, separate, cook, and chill. See part IV, "Play it Safe With Food," on page 239, for details on each step, as well as proper temperatures to keep food safe when you store it, thaw it, prepare it, cook it, serve it, and save leftovers. Older adults should be particularly careful.

In addition, older adults need to avoid eating or drinking raw (unpasteurized) milk or any products made from unpasteurized milk, raw or partially cooked eggs or foods containing raw eggs, raw or undercooked meat and poultry, raw or undercooked fish or shellfish, unpasteurized juices, and raw sprouts.

Bringing it together

We've talked a lot about the healthy eating plan: getting a variety of fruits, vegetables, whole grains, and fat-free or low-fat milk and equivalent milk products; including lean meats, poultry, fish, legumes (dry beans and peas), eggs, nuts, and seeds; and balancing calorie intake with calorie needs. Each major food group provides a variety of nutrients, so it's important to include all food groups in your daily eating plan.

MY JOURNEY TO LIVING A HEALTHIER LIFESTYLE

by Regina D. Coles from Atlanta, Georgia

At the age of forty, my health was something that I took for granted. I was 165 pounds and I wore a size 16. I was eating whatever I wanted to eat without any thought of how my eating habits were affecting my health. I failed to get regular physical exams during this time because I felt fine and I saw no reason to schedule regular doctor's office visits. However, all of that changed with an office visit that I scheduled with a new physician. He explained to me what cholesterol and heart disease were, as well as other health problems that develop as we age.

My test results indicated a cholesterol level of 304, and my blood pressure was elevated as well as my sugar level. I was shocked to learn that all of this was going on at the same time, and I was determined that I was going to follow the

(continued)

MY JOURNEY TO LIVING A HEALTHIER LIFESTYLE
(continued)

lifestyle changes that my doctor recommended. He added that making these changes would lead to a healthier and happier way of living. My doctor advised me to begin an exercise program that I could enjoy so that I could remain motivated enough to stick with it. The next day, I began to run on a nearby high school track. When I first began, I ran only as far as I felt comfortable running, then I would stop and start to walk. I gradually increased my distance to 3 miles. I always made sure that I had plenty of water to drink after my run.

The next change I had to make was my diet. When my doctor explained the changes that I had to make, I thought he was joking. It turns out that he was quite serious. He recommended chicken and fish, which had to be broiled or baked without the skin. I could eat lean cuts of beef twice a week prepared the same way as the skinless chicken and fish. I also had to learn to eliminate some of the fat from my foods. I became conscious of how much fat I was consuming. I also began to read the labels on the food I bought and began making better choices.

Of course, I complained because I missed my old way of preparing my meals. You see, I loved fried fish and chicken and fresh collards, turnips, cabbage, and green beans prepared with salt pork. I must admit that I was truly amazed when, at the end of 6 weeks, I noticed that I was actually losing weight as a result of my lifestyle change.

I realized 6 months later that this new lifestyle change would become a permanent way of living because one of the benefits was my changed attitude toward life. I began to develop a positive attitude toward life. I also became more outgoing and ready to face new challenges.

After 1 year, my blood pressure drastically declined and so did my sugar level. My weight returned to normal, and I learned to enjoy my new way of eating. I looked and felt younger, and I noticed that I had more energy. Of course, I've faced some illnesses along the way, some more serious than others. Last year, I experienced an illness that was potentially fatal. I was told by my doctor that my survival was possibly due to the diet and exercise changes that I had made many years ago and maintained throughout the years.

By the time I became an older American, I was celebrating a new body with a transformed mind. I feel that the changes that I was determined to make in my younger years have greatly affected my health and appearance today. Thanks to the lifestyle changes that I made nearly 30 years ago, today I feel great and I am blessed to be an active, healthy, and productive older American.

For older adults, every day it's important to eat:

- fiber-containing foods
- vitamin B_{12}-fortified foods, such as fortified cereals, or take the crystalline form of vitamin B_{12} supplements
- vitamin D-fortified foods, such as fortified milk or orange juice, which are important for calcium absorption and can reduce the risk of bone loss.

In general, older adults should get enough foods that contain calcium, potassium, fiber, magnesium, and vitamins A, C, D, and E, without eating too many foods high in calories, saturated and *trans* fats, cholesterol, added sugars, and salt (sodium).

We've already talked about some adjustments to make to our diets. Now, let's quickly review how this fits into your daily calorie needs based on "My Personal Profile," or if you are caring for older adults, take a moment to figure out their range.

Special Considerations

For those of you 65 years of age and older, there are some important things to consider when it comes to physical activity:

- The most important thing to do is to become less sedentary.
- Use a gradual or stepwise approach.
- Focus more on moderate activity than achieving high levels of activity.
- Try to spend time on both strength training and cardio or aerobic activities, rather than just focusing on one or the other.
- Perform balance exercises to reduce your risk of fall and injury.
- To maintain the range of motion necessary for daily activities, perform activities that maintain or increase flexibility.

Good to do: If you have a chronic condition, manage your risk of injury by working with a health care provider to develop an activity plan.

For example, a 60-year-old, sedentary woman should aim for 1,600 calories per day, while a 60-year-old, sedentary male should aim for 2,000 calories per day.

		Activity Level		
		Sedentary	Moderately Active	Active
Gender	Age (years)	Calorie		
Female	51+	1,600	1,800	2,000–2,200
Male	51+	2,000	2,200–2,400	2,400–2,800

When increasing the amount of fruits, vegetables, and legumes you eat, be sure to eat them in place of less nutritious foods, not in addition to them, if weight control is part of your goal. Next, let's work in some physical activity.

You can! Be active.

Many older adults may feel that they are too tired to be physically active or that they have earned their rest. However, physical activity is a critical part of a healthy lifestyle, and for older adults, physical activity may take on even more meaning. Continuing to live independently—doing the things that you enjoy— can be linked to being active. Increasing your heartbeat, strengthening your muscles, and increasing your flexibility contribute to physical fitness and the ability to do everyday activities like climbing the stairs, shopping for groceries, and visiting with family and friends.

> "Physical activity is like a savings account. The more you put in, the more you get out of it!"
>
> — Earl, age 62

Older adults may want to consult with their health care provider, if they have certain chronic diseases or are taking medications, before starting vigorous physical activity. Let's also clear up a misconception—that older adults should not participate in physical activity because of a risk of falls or injury. Actually, the opposite is true. Sedentary older adults have a higher risk of falls and regular physical activity may reduce their risk. Research also shows that regular physical activity can promote psychological well-being and can aid in reducing feelings of mild-to-moderate depression and anxiety. On a day that you're feeling a bit tired, down, or stressed, consider taking a brisk walk around your neighborhood or at the mall. Start small, have a positive attitude, build up to more vigorous activities, and continue to enjoy all that life has to offer you!

Let's get into the nitty gritty…for adults ages 65 and older, here's what science tells us to do:

- At a minimum, do moderately-intense cardio or aerobic activity for at least 30 minutes per day, most days of the week.

AND

- At a minimum, do strength-training exercises, 2 days per week.

Moderate activity: Intensity is relative to your level of fitness. For some older adults, moderately-intense physical activities include:

- walking briskly
- biking at a casual pace
- dancing (ballroom, line dancing, jazz, or tap)
- water aerobics
- golfing without a cart
- light gardening/yard work such as raking or pushing a power lawn mower
- actively playing with children
- doubles tennis.

Vigorous activity: For some older adults, vigorously-intense physical activities include:

- jogging
- swimming laps
- singles tennis
- heavy yard work.

What is strength training and why do it?

We talked about this in chapter 10, "Making Physical Activity Part of a Healthier You," because it's important for all adults regardless of age. But it's worth repeating. Strength-training exercises are resistance exercises that increase the strength of your muscles, help maintain the integrity of your bones, and may improve your balance, coordination, and mobility. Both strength training and cardio or aerobic activities are important. In particular, strength training helps develop and maintain a healthy skeleton and muscle mass.

A few examples of strength-training exercises are:

- digging in a garden
- chopping wood
- using a push lawn mower
- bicep curls
- yoga (some types are more strengthening than others)
- leg lifts
- squats.

What is balance training? Some exercises improve your balance and strength at the same time. If you are at risk of falling, you should include balance exercises as part of your strength-training activities. Some examples include:

- rising up and down on your toes while standing and holding a stable chair or countertop
- walking a straight line heel to toe
- side leg raises while standing and holding onto a chair
- knee flexions (while standing and holding onto a chair, bend knee so your foot lifts behind you)
- hip flexions (while standing and holding onto a chair, raise knee toward chest).

Remember: You can do it. It's time well spent to help give you more time, extra quality years to spend with your family and friends enjoying life!

Chapter 12. Healthier Children

Many of us touch the lives of children in some way. We have an opportunity to give children the building blocks they need to lead a healthy lifestyle. As parents, doctors, educators, extended family, or friends—we are all in a position to set good examples. By teaching children the importance of good nutrition and regular physical activity early, they'll learn good habits to last a lifetime. Whether it's a family effort or simply taking advantage of the time spent with children, healthy choices start with all of us.

Since children are growing, sometimes it's hard to know their weight status—are they overweight or will they "grow" out of it? We know that maintaining a healthy weight throughout childhood and adolescence may reduce the risk of becoming an overweight or obese adult. Just as you determined your own Body Mass Index (BMI) in chapter 4, "Where to Start," the same can be done for children and adolescents. However, their BMI is age- and gender-specific using growth curve charts. You can get an idea of the weight status of your child by looking at the growth chart for boys 2 to 20 years in part V, "Dietary Guidelines for Americans, 2005," figure 3, on page 275, or at: www.cdc.gov/growthcharts for additional growth charts. This is best done with the help of your child's doctor.

Always check with your child's health care provider about your child's rate of growth and development before starting him or her on any type of weight-gain or weight-loss diet. A health care provider can give you good nutrition and weight management approaches that take into consideration that your child is growing and developing. This is especially important if your child has a medical condition or is on medication.

For children 2+

The keys to healthy eating are variety, balance, and moderation. Just as you determined the amount of food from each food group that was right for you, children and adolescents have amounts that are right for them, too. You can estimate the amount of calories your child should be eating each day as you did for yourself. Turn to page 16 in chapter 4, "Where to Start," and compare your child's age and gender with his or her activity level to determine the approximate number of calories she or he should be eating each day. Then, you can look at the eating plans in appendix A, on page 320, and choose one that fits your child's calorie needs. Be sure to check with your doctor to get his or her advice before you make any specific changes.

Here are some additional considerations to take when finding a healthy eating plan for your child.

Whole grains: Everyone, including kids, should consume whole-grain products often, and at least half the grains they eat should be whole grains. Think whole-grain cereals and sandwiches made with whole wheat bread, but be sure to check the ingredient list for "whole wheat."

Calcium: Because calcium is important for growing bones, children 2 to 8 years should consume 2 cups per day of fat-free or low-fat milk or equivalent milk products. Children 9 years and older should consume 3 cups per day of fat-free or low-fat milk or equivalent milk products.

Fruits and vegetables: The number of fruits and vegetables children should eat is determined by their calorie needs. Figure this out the same way you did for yourself. First, estimate your child's activity level and compare that to the table found on page 16 in chapter 4, "Where to Start." From there, you'll be able to determine how many calories your child should be eating, along with what is the best healthy eating pattern to follow—including the right number of fruits and vegetables. (See appendix A, on page 320, for Eating Patterns.)

Fats and salt: It's important for us to know how much total fat and the types of fat we eat (for example, saturated and *trans* fats) and the same holds true for children. When kids reach 2 years, it is time to start watching the types of fat and how much salt they eat. Children who eat high saturated fats or salt (sodium) diets can be at risk of high blood cholesterol and high blood pressure just like adults. That's why total fat intake should be kept between 30 and 35 percent of calories for children ages 2 to 3 years, and between 25 and 35 percent of calories for children and adolescents ages 4 to 18. Most fats should come from sources of polyunsaturated and monounsaturated fatty acids, such as fish, nuts, and vegetable oils. Following the eating plans, at the calorie needs for your children, will help them get the nutrients they need to grow up healthy.

Cavity (caries) prevention: Consider how many sugary snacks (think cavities!) your children are eating. Sugary snacks contain calories, but few or no essential nutrients, and may increase the chance that your kids will get cavities. Some helpful tips to reduce cavities: regular brushing, fluoride toothpaste, and fluoridated water. Also replace sugary snacks with healthy snacks—fruits, vegetables, and whole grains can make a difference.

Food safety: In addition to the general food safety precautions you'll find in this book, there are a couple of special considerations when it comes to children and food safety. Infants and young children should not eat or drink raw (unpasteurized) milk or any products made from unpasteurized milk, raw or partially cooked eggs or foods containing raw eggs, raw or undercooked meat and poultry, raw or under-cooked fish or shellfish, unpasteurized juices, and raw sprouts. (For more information, visit www.cfsan.fda.gov.)

CARLOS IS A STAR!

I'm Carlos's mom. My son is a fifth grader and doing well at school. He loves soccer—his room is covered with posters of his favorite team and his idol, David Beckham. He comes straight home from school every day and does his home-work. Good, I thought? A couple of weeks ago, I asked him about soccer. He looked at me with tears and said, "The kids play soccer after school, but I never get picked. They all run faster than me and I get tired—I can't keep up. Some of them teased me saying that I'm too fat." It just hurts me to see him so down on himself. He's such a good kid.

I wanted to do something. I took him to the pediatrician for a checkup. The pe-diatrician examined Carlos and asked him how he was and a lot of questions about what he eats—sodas, french fries, other stuff...and what he likes to do—it was clear that the issue was Carlos's weight. Our pediatrician reassured him that we could work on this together—including me! The pediatrician told us that overall, Carlos was healthy and would grow more, and that would help a lot. But he also explained that it would be helpful if Carlos paid more attention to what he was eating each day. The pediatrician emphasized, eyeing me—that it would be a good idea if the whole family tried to eat better as well—more fruits and vegetables...and low-fat milk instead of sugar sodas.

We started grocery shopping together so Carlos could pick out foods he liked and that are good for all of us. The pediatrician said Carlos needs at least 60 minutes of physical activity most days of the week, so we tried to come up with things to do each day—we kept a list in the kitchen for the entire week. It was hard at first, but now, Carlos is playing more and says he feels like he has more energy—and so does the whole family.

Yesterday, Carlos kicked his first field goal! His buddies jumped all over him. Carlos may not be a soccer star yet, but he's my star! Just hearing him talk about his goal—and even seeing him head out the door to play in the afternoon, is worth it all.

A smart start

We've all had to balance, at one time or another, what children want with what's best for them. Nobody wants to feel like they are denying a child certain types of food. Making smart choices doesn't have to come down to this. Here are some tips and strategies that might help reach a healthy balance:

- Try to keep track of children's meal/snack and physical activity patterns so you can encourage a healthful lifestyle.
- For younger children, the family setting is a good place to encourage them (along with the rest of the family) to eat a variety of differently colored vegetables and fruits each day. You can start their day with 100% fruit or vegetable juice. Slice fruit on top of a whole-grain cereal. Serve a salad with lunch and an apple as an afternoon snack. Include vegetables with dinner.
- Remember: Fill your shopping cart with fruits, vegetables, nuts, and fat-free or low-fat milk and limit candy, soft drinks, chips, and cookies. Children will soon learn to make these types of smart food choices outside the home as well.
- Choose a variety of foods. No single food or food group supplies all the nutrients in the amounts that you need for good health. If you plan for pizza one night, include other food or food groups by adding a salad, serving fat-free or low-fat milk, and having fruit for dessert.

Eat smart.

Eating together is an ideal way for family and friends to spend time together and enjoy each other's company. Whether you're eating at home or eating out on the go, it's important to eat smart. Check off some of the tips you can easily put into action. Try one or two at a time. Don't bite off more than you can chew!

- Be consistent. Establish a family meal routine, and set times for breakfast, lunch, dinner, and snacks. Eat together whenever possible.
- Take charge of the foods children eat. When you serve a meal, a child can choose to eat it or not; but don't offer to substitute a less healthy alternative when the child refuses to eat what you've served.
- Limit children's access to the refrigerator and snack cupboards.
- Turn off the TV during meals, and limit children's snacking when watching TV. It is easy to lose track of how much they are eating, especially if the snack is a bag of pretzels instead of a small bowl.
- Serve a vegetable or fruit with every meal and at snack time.

- Reward children with praise and fun activities rather than food.
- Involve children in meal planning and food preparation. They are more likely to eat what they help to make.
- While shopping and cooking, teach children about the food groups and the importance of a healthy eating plan. Throughout the day, help them choose the types and amounts of foods they need from the different food groups.
- Teach children how to read food labels and use the quick guide to the percent Daily Value (% DV): 5% DV or less is low; 20% DV or more is high.
- Use low-fat cooking methods such as baking, roasting, and grilling; and when you use oil, select those such as olive or canola oils.
- Serve water and fat-free or low-fat milk, with and between meals. Children over 2 years should be encouraged to drink fat-free or low-fat milk. Whole milk is recommended for children from 1 to 2 years old. Check with your health care provider for feeding recommendations for younger children and those with special needs.
- Teach children how to make wise food choices away from home—at school cafeterias, restaurants, and vending machines.
- Teach children to pay attention to both the quality and quantity of their food choices. More food is not always better; they need to understand appropriate portion sizes.

Good nutrition and regular physical activity should be part of an overall healthy lifestyle. To grow healthfully, children must balance the calories they eat with what they use up being physically active.

Play time can be physical activity time.

Play is an important part of growing and developing. It allows children to learn, explore, and be physically active. All of this is critical for children to help strengthen muscles, bones, and joints, and it gives them the opportunity to gain confidence while having fun! Children need to get at least 60 minutes of physical activity on most, if not all, days of the week. Playing hopscotch, tossing a ball back and forth, and dancing, in addition to organized sports, are some good ways for your child to be active and learn important life skills along the way.

Some examples of activities listed by intensity of physical activity (see box). Your children can always step up the intensity by working harder!

Moderate	Vigorous
Light yard work	Running
Walking	Swimming
Bicycling	Basketball

- Be a physically active role model and have fun with children. Since adults need 30 minutes of daily physical activity, play together! Then, make sure the child gets in another 30 minutes for a total of 60. Another 30 minutes is probably good for you, too.
- Walk with children at every available opportunity—if possible to school or to the store on errands. Take a walk with family or friends after dinner instead of watching TV or playing computer games.
- Plan active weekends. Include biking, hiking, skating, walking, or playing ball. Take a trip to the park, swimming pool, or ice skating rink. If you work on weekends, arrange a physically active play date for your child.
- Offer to join children in their favorite physical activities, or enroll children in a group exercise program.
- Include children in active chores such as dog walking, house cleaning, car washing, and yard work.
- Limit physically inactive behavior such as TV watching and computer time.
- Avoid using TV as a child-sitter or pacifier. Offer active alternatives to screen time—jumping rope, playing hide-and-seek, or running an errand. Children love it when you are active with them and share in what they do.
- Keep TVs out of children's rooms.
- Give your children gifts that encourage physical activity—active games or sporting equipment.
- Talk with your schools about ways to incorporate non-competitive physical activity during the day.

An easy and fun way to keep children active and eating right is to create a weekly calendar of healthy lifestyle activities. Use some of the ideas in this chapter to start building a healthy family (or "friends") plan that works for everyone's schedule. Let everyone choose a weekly activity and take charge of it. Also, check out the kid-friendly recipes in part IV, "Recipes and Resources," to help empower children to prepare their own foods, with adult supervision, of course!

Part III

Making a Healthier You Happen—
Worksheets

My Personal Profile

My Healthy Eating Plan Using the
DASH Eating Plan

One Week With the DASH Eating Plan

My Shopping List

Tips for Healthy Substitutes

Tips for Using the Food Label

My Physical Activity Tracker

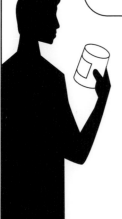

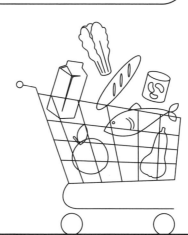

My Personal Profile

Name: _____

Today's date: _____

Age: _____

Height (in.): _____

Weight (lb.): _____ Waist size (in.): _____

BMI: Use the BMI chart on page 12 or use this equation:

$$\frac{\text{wt (lb.)}}{\text{Height (in.) x height (in.)}} \times 703 = \underline{\hspace{5cm}}$$

BMI ranges:
- < 18.5 = underweight
- 18.5–24.9 = normal weight
- 25–29.9 = overweight
- > 30 = obese

My BMI indicates that I am: (Please circle)
underweight   normal weight   overweight   obese

My risk factors are: (Please circle)
- high blood pressure (hypertension)
- high LDL cholesterol ("bad" cholesterol)
- low HDL cholesterol ("good" cholesterol)
- high triglycerides
- high blood glucose (sugar)
- family history of premature heart disease
- physical inactivity
- cigarette smoking

My physical activity level is: (Please circle)
sedentary   moderately active   active

- *Sedentary* means a lifestyle that includes only the light physical activity associated with typical day-to-day life.
- *Moderately* active means a lifestyle that includes physical activity equivalent to walking about 1.5 to 3 miles per day at 3 to 4 miles per hour, in addition to the light physical activity associated with typical day-to-day life.
- *Active* means a lifestyle that includes physical activity equivalent to walking more than 3 miles per day at 3 to 4 miles per hour, in addition to the light physical activity associated with typical day-to-day life.

A healthy weight range for my height is: (Based on the BMI chart) _____

Estimated daily calorie needs, my goal: _____

My Healthy Eating Plan Using the DASH Eating Plan

Food	Amount (serving size)	Sodium (mg)	Grains	Vegetables	Fruits	Milk products	Meats, fish, and poultry	Nuts, seeds, and legumes	Fats and oils	Sweets and added sugars
Number of Servings by Food Group:										
Breakfast Example: whole wheat bread, with soft margarine	2 slices 2 tsp	299 102	2						2	
Lunch										
Dinner										
Snacks										
Totals										
Compare yours with the DASH Eating Plan										
Read food labels to compare the sodium content of foods. See page 57 to learn how to find sodium information on food labels.										

Use information from appendix A-1 to find meal plans for your calorie level.

My Healthy Eating Plan Using the DASH Eating Plan

Food	Amount (serving size)	Sodium (mg)	Grains	Vegetables	Fruits	Milk products	Meats, fish, and poultry	Nuts, seeds, and legumes	Fats and oils	Sweets and added sugars
Number of Servings by Food Group:										
Breakfast										
Lunch										
Dinner										
Snacks										
Totals										
Compare yours with the DASH Eating Plan										

Read food labels to compare the sodium content of foods. See page 57 to learn how to find sodium information on food labels.

Use information from appendix A-1 to find meal plans for your calorie level.

My Healthy Eating Plan Using the DASH Eating Plan

Food	Amount (serving size)	Sodium (mg)	Grains	Vegetables	Fruits	Milk products	Meats, fish, and poultry	Nuts, seeds, and legumes	Fats and oils	Sweets and added sugars
Number of Servings by Food Group:										
Breakfast										
Lunch										
Dinner										
Snacks										
Totals										
Compare yours with the DASH Eating Plan										
Read food labels to compare the sodium content of foods. See page 57 to learn how to find sodium information on food labels.										

Use information from appendix A-1 to find meal plans for your calorie level.

My Healthy Eating Plan Using the DASH Eating Plan

Food	Amount (serving size)	Sodium (mg)	Grains	Vegetables	Fruits	Milk products	Meats, fish, and poultry	Nuts, seeds, and legumes	Fats and oils	Sweets and added sugars
Number of Servings by Food Group:										
Breakfast										
Lunch										
Dinner										
Snacks										
Totals										
Compare yours with the DASH Eating Plan										

Read food labels to compare the sodium content of foods. See page 57 to learn how to find sodium information on food labels.

Use information from appendix A-1 to find meal plans for your calorie level.

My Healthy Eating Plan Using the DASH Eating Plan

Food	Amount (serving size)	Sodium (mg)	Grains	Vegetables	Fruits	Milk products	Meats, fish, and poultry	Nuts, seeds, and legumes	Fats and oils	Sweets and added sugars
Number of Servings by Food Group:										
Breakfast										
Lunch										
Dinner										
Snacks										
Totals										
Compare yours with the DASH Eating Plan										
Read food labels to compare the sodium content of foods. See page 57 to learn how to find sodium information on food labels.										

Use information from appendix A-1 to find meal plans for your calorie level.

My Healthy Eating Plan Using the DASH Eating Plan

Food	Amount (serving size)	Sodium (mg)	Grains	Vegetables	Fruits	Milk products	Meats, fish, and poultry	Nuts, seeds, and legumes	Fats and oils	Sweets and added sugars
Number of Servings by Food Group:										
Breakfast										
Lunch										
Dinner										
Snacks										
Totals										
Compare yours with the DASH Eating Plan										

Read food labels to compare the sodium content of foods. See page 57 to learn how to find sodium information on food labels.

Use information from appendix A-1 to find meal plans for your calorie level.

My Healthy Eating Plan Using the DASH Eating Plan

Food	Amount (serving size)	Sodium (mg)	Grains	Vegetables	Fruits	Milk products	Meats, fish, and poultry	Nuts, seeds, and legumes	Fats and oils	Sweets and added sugars
Number of Servings by Food Group:										
Breakfast										
Lunch										
Dinner										
Snacks										
Totals										
Compare yours with the DASH Eating Plan										
Read food labels to compare the sodium content of foods. See page 57 to learn how to find sodium information on food labels.										

Use information from appendix A-1 to find meal plans for your calorie level.

One Week With the DASH Eating Plan

(2,000 calories)

Day 1   Number of Servings by DASH Food Group

2,300-mg Sodium (Na) Menu	Na (mg)	Grains	Vegetables	Fruits	Milk products	Meats, fish, and poultry	Nuts, seeds, and legumes	Fats and oils	Sweets and added sugars
Breakfast									
³/₄ cup bran flakes cereal:	220	1							
1 medium banana	1			1					
1 cup milk, low-fat	107				1				
1 slice whole wheat bread:	149	1							
1 tsp soft (tub) margarine	26							1	
1 cup orange juice	5			2					
Lunch									
³/₄ cup chicken salad*:	179					1		1	
2 slices whole wheat bread	299	2							
1 Tbsp Dijon mustard	373								
salad:									
¹/₂ cup fresh cucumber slices	1		1						
¹/₂ cup tomato wedges	5		1						
1 Tbsp sunflower seeds	0						¹/₂		
1 tsp Italian dressing, reduced calorie	43								
¹/₂ cup fruit cocktail, juice pack	5			1					
Dinner									
3 oz beef, eye of the round:	35					1			
2 Tbsp beef gravy, fat-free	165								
1 cup green beans, sautéed with:	12		2						
¹/₂ tsp canola oil	0							¹/₂	
1 small baked potato:	14		1						
1 Tbsp sour cream, fat-free	21								
1 Tbsp grated cheddar cheese, natural, reduced fat	67								
1 Tbsp chopped scallions	1								
1 small whole wheat roll:	148	1							
1 tsp soft (tub) margarine	26							1	
1 small apple	1			1					
1 cup milk, low-fat	107				1				
Snacks									
¹/₃ cup almonds, unsalted	0						1		
¹/₄ cup raisins	4			1					
¹/₂ cup fruit yogurt, fat-free, no sugar added	86				¹/₂				
Totals	**2,101**	**5**	**5**	**6**	**2¹/₂**	**2**	**1¹/₂**	**3¹/₂**	**0**

Nutrients Per Day

Calories: 2,062	**Carbohydrate:** 284 g
Total fat: 63 g	**Protein:** 114 g
Calories from fat: 28%	**Calcium:** 1,220 mg
Saturated fat: 13 g	**Magnesium:** 594 mg
Calories from saturated fat: 6%	**Potassium:** 4,909 mg
Cholesterol: 155 mg	**Fiber:** 37 g
Sodium: 2,101 mg	

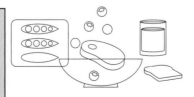

*recipe on page 144

Day 2 / 2,300-mg Sodium (Na) Menu	Na (mg)	Grains	Vegetables	Fruits	Milk products	Meats, fish, and poultry	Nuts, seeds, and legumes	Fats and oils	Sweets and added sugars
Breakfast									
1/2 cup instant oatmeal	54	1							
1 mini whole wheat bagel:	84	1							
1 Tbsp peanut butter	81						1/2		
1 medium banana	1			1					
1 cup milk, low-fat	107				1				
Lunch									
chicken breast sandwich:									
2 slices (3 oz) chicken breast, skinless	65					1			
2 slices whole wheat bread	299	2							
1 slice (3/4 oz) cheddar cheese, natural, reduced fat	202				1/2				
1 large leaf romaine lettuce	1		1/4						
2 slices tomato	2		1/2						
1 Tbsp mayonnaise, low-fat	101							1	
1 cup cantaloupe	26			2					
1 cup apple juice	21			2					
Dinner									
1 cup spaghetti:	1	2							
3/4 cup vegetarian spaghetti sauce*	479		1 1/2						
3 Tbsp Parmesan cheese	287				1/2				
spinach salad:									
1 cup fresh spinach leaves	24		1						
1/4 cup fresh carrots, grated	19		1/2						
1/4 cup fresh mushrooms, sliced	1		1/2						
1 Tbsp vinaigrette salad dressing**	0							1/2	
1/2 cup corn, cooked from frozen	1		1						
1/2 cup canned pears, juice pack	5			1					
Snacks									
1/3 cup almonds	0						1		
1/4 cup dried apricots	3			1					
1 cup fruit yogurt, fat-free, no sugar added	173				1				
Totals	2,035	6	5 1/4	7	3	1	1 1/2	1 1/2	0

Number of Servings by DASH Food Group

Nutrients Per Day

Calories: 2,027	Carbohydrate: 288 g
Total fat: 64 g	Protein: 99 g
Calories from fat: 28%	Calcium: 1,370 mg
Saturated fat: 13 g	Magnesium: 535 mg
Calories from saturated fat: 6%	Potassium: 4,715 mg
Cholesterol: 114 mg	Fiber: 34 g
Sodium: 2,035 mg	

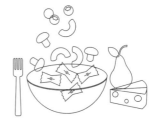

*recipe on page 196
**recipe on page 129

| Day 3 | | | Number of Servings by DASH Food Group | | | | | | |

2,300-mg Sodium (Na) Menu	Na (mg)	Grains	Vegetables	Fruits	Milk products	Meats, fish, and poultry	Nuts, seeds, and legumes	Fats and oils	Sweets and added sugars
Breakfast									
3/4 cup bran flakes cereal:	220	1							
1 medium banana	1			1					
1 cup milk, low-fat	107				1				
1 slice whole wheat bread:	149	1							
1 tsp soft (tub) margarine	26							1	
1 cup orange juice	6			2					
Lunch									
beef barbecue sandwich:									
2 oz beef, eye of round	26					2/3			
1 Tbsp barbecue sauce	156								
2 slices (1 1/2 oz) cheddar cheese, natural, reduced fat	405				1				
1 hamburger bun	183	2							
1 large leaf romaine lettuce	1		1/4						
2 slices tomato	2		1/2						
1 cup new potato salad*	17		2						
1 medium orange	0			1					
Dinner									
3 oz cod:	70					1			
1 tsp lemon juice	1								
1/2 cup brown rice	5	1							
1 cup spinach, cooked from frozen, sautéed with:	184		2						
1 tsp canola oil	0							1	
1 Tbsp almonds, slivered	0						1/4		
1 small cornbread muffin, made with oil:	119	1							
1 tsp soft (tub) margarine	26							1	
Snacks									
1 cup fruit yogurt, fat-free, no added sugar:	173				1				
1 Tbsp sunflower seeds, unsalted	0						1/2		
2 large graham cracker rectangles:	156	1							
1 Tbsp peanut butter	81						1/2		
Totals	**2,114**	**7**	**4 3/4**	**4**	**3**	**1 2/3**	**1 1/4**	**3**	**0**

Nutrients Per Day

Calories: 1,997	Carbohydrate: 289 g
Total fat: 56 g	Protein: 103 g
Calories from fat: 25%	Calcium: 1,537 mg
Saturated fat: 12 g	Magnesium: 630 mg
Calories from saturated fat: 6%	Potassium: 4,676 mg
Cholesterol: 140 mg	Fiber: 34 g
Sodium: 2,114 mg	

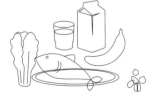

*recipe on page 209

Day 4 — Number of Servings by DASH Food Group

2,300-mg Sodium (Na) Menu	Na (mg)	Grains	Vegetables	Fruits	Milk products	Meats, fish, and poultry	Nuts, seeds, and legumes	Fats and oils	Sweets and added sugars
Breakfast									
1 slice whole wheat bread:	149	1							
1 tsp soft (tub) margarine	26							1	
1 cup fruit yogurt, fat-free, no added sugar	173				1				
1 medium peach	0			1					
1/2 cup grape juice	4			1					
Lunch									
ham and cheese sandwich:									
2 oz ham, low-fat, low-sodium	549					2/3			
1 slice (3/4 oz) cheddar cheese, natural, reduced fat	202				1/2				
2 slices whole wheat bread	299	2							
1 large leaf romaine lettuce	1		1/4						
2 slices tomato	2		1/2						
1 Tbsp mayonnaise, low-fat	101							1	
1 carrot sticks	84		2						
Dinner									
chicken and Spanish rice*	341	1				1			
1 cup green peas, sautéed with:	115		2						
1 tsp canola oil	0							1	
1 cup cantaloupe chunks	26			2					
1 cup milk, low-fat	107				1				
Snacks									
1/3 cup almonds	0						1		
1 cup apple juice	21			2					
1/4 cup apricots	3			1					
1 cup milk, low-fat	107				1				
Totals	**2,312**	**4**	**4 3/4**	**7**	**3 1/2**	**1 2/3**	**1**	**3**	**0**

Nutrients Per Day

Calories: 2,024	Carbohydrate: 279 g
Total fat: 59 g	Protein: 110 g
Calories from fat: 26%	Calcium: 1,417 mg
Saturated fat: 12 g	Magnesium: 538 mg
Calories from saturated fat: 5%	Potassium: 4,575 mg
Cholesterol: 148 mg	Fiber: 35 g
Sodium: 2,312 mg	

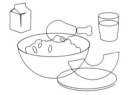

*recipe on page 171

Day 5   Number of Servings by DASH Food Group

2,300-mg Sodium (Na) Menu	Na (mg)	Grains	Vegetables	Fruits	Milk products	Meats, fish, and poultry	Nuts, seeds, and legumes	Fats and oils	Sweets and added sugars
Breakfast									
1 cup whole-grain oat rings cereal:	273	1							
1 medium banana	1			1					
1 cup milk, low-fat	107				1				
1 medium raisin bagel:	272	2							
1 Tbsp peanut butter	81						1/2		
1 cup orange juice	5			2					
Lunch									
tuna salad plate:									
1/2 cup tuna salad*	171					1			
1 large leaf romaine lettuce	1		1/4						
1 slice whole wheat bread	149	1							
cucumber salad:									
1 cup fresh cucumber slices	2		2						
1/2 cup tomato wedges	5		1						
1 Tbsp vinaigrette dressing	133							1	
1/2 cup cottage cheese, low-fat:	459				1/4				
1/2 cup canned pineapple, juice pack	1			1					
1 Tbsp almonds	0						1/4		
Dinner									
3 oz turkey meatloaf**	205					1			
1 small baked potato:	14		1						
1 Tbsp sour cream, fat-free	21								
1 Tbsp cheddar cheese, natural, reduced fat, grated	67								
1 scallion stalk, chopped	1								
1 cup collard greens, sautéed with:	85		2						
1 tsp canola oil	0							1	
1 small whole wheat roll	148	1							
1 medium peach	0			1					
Snacks									
1 cup fruit yogurt, fat-free, no added sugar	173				1				
2 Tbsp sunflower seeds	0						1		
Totals	**2,373**	**5**	**6 1/4**	**5**	**2 1/4**	**2**	**1 3/4**	**2**	**0**

Nutrients Per Day

Calories: 1,976
Total fat: 57 g
Calories from fat: 26%
Saturated fat: 11 g
Calories from saturated fat: 5%
Cholesterol: 158 mg
Sodium: 2,373 mg

Carbohydrate: 275 g
Protein: 111 g
Calcium: 1,470 mg
Magnesium: 495 mg
Potassium: 4,769 mg
Fiber: 30 g

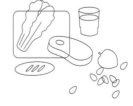

*recipe on page 149
**recipe on page 182

Day 6 — Number of Servings by DASH Food Group

2,300-mg Sodium (Na) Menu	Na (mg)	Grains	Vegetables	Fruits	Milk products	Meats, fish, and poultry	Nuts, seeds, and legumes	Fats and oils	Sweets and added sugars
Breakfast									
1 granola bar, low-fat	81	1							
1 medium banana	1			1					
1/2 cup fruit yogurt, fat-free, no sugar added	86				1/2				
1 cup orange juice	5			2					
1 cup milk, low-fat	107				1				
Lunch									
turkey breast sandwich:									
3 oz turkey breast	48					1			
2 slices whole wheat bread	299	2							
1 large leaf romaine lettuce	1		1/4						
2 slices tomato	2		1/2						
2 tsp mayonnaise, low-fat	67							2/3	
1 Tbsp Dijon mustard	373								
1 cup steamed broccoli, cooked from frozen	11		2						
1 medium orange	0			1					
Dinner									
3 oz spicy baked fish*	50					1			
1 cup scallion rice**	18	2							
spinach sauté:									
1/2 cup spinach, cooked from frozen	92		1						
2 tsp canola oil	0							2	
1 Tbsp almonds, slivered	0						1/4		
1 cup carrots, cooked from frozen	84		2						
1 small whole wheat roll:	148	1							
1 tsp soft (tub) margarine	26							1	
1 small cookie	60								1
Snacks									
2 Tbsp peanuts, unsalted	1						1/2		
1 cup milk, low-fat	107				1				
1/4 cup dried apricots	3			1					
Totals	1,671	6	5 3/4	5	2 1/2	2	3/4	3 2/3	1

Nutrients Per Day

Calories: 1,939	Carbohydrate: 268 g
Total fat: 58 g	Protein: 105 g
Calories from fat: 27%	Calcium: 1,210 mg
Saturated fat: 12 g	Magnesium: 548 mg
Calories from saturated fat: 6%	Potassium: 4,710 mg
Cholesterol: 171 mg	Fiber: 36 g
Sodium: 1,671 mg	

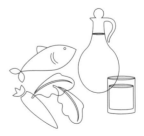

*recipe on page 188
**recipe on page 205

| Day 7 | Number of Servings by DASH Food Group | | | | | | | | |

2,300-mg Sodium (Na) Menu	Na (mg)	Grains	Vegetables	Fruits	Milk products	Meats, fish, and poultry	Nuts, seeds, and legumes	Fats and oils	Sweets and added sugars
Breakfast									
1 cup whole-grain oat rings cereal:	273	1							
1 medium banana	1			1					
1 cup milk, low-fat	107				1				
1 cup fruit yogurt, fat-free, no sugar added	173				1				
Lunch									
tuna salad sandwich:									
¹/₂ cup tuna, drained, rinsed	39					1			
1 Tbsp mayonnaise, low-fat	101							1	
1 large leaf romaine lettuce	1		¹/₄						
2 slices tomato	2		¹/₂						
2 slices whole wheat bread	299	2							
1 medium apple	1			1					
1 cup milk, low-fat	107				1				
Dinner									
¹/₆ recipe zucchini lasagna*	368	3	1		1				
salad:									
1 cup fresh spinach leaves	24		1						
1 cup tomato wedges	9		2						
2 Tbsp croutons, seasoned	62	¹/₄							
1 Tbsp vinaigrette dressing, reduced calorie	133							¹/₂	
1 Tbsp sunflower seeds	0						¹/₂		
1 small whole wheat roll:	148	1							
1 tsp soft (tub) margarine	45							1	
1 cup grape juice	8			2					
Snacks									
¹/₃ cup almonds, unsalted	0						1		
¹/₄ cup dry apricots	3			1					
6 whole wheat crackers	166	1							
Totals	2,069	8¹/₄	4³/₄	5	4	1	1¹/₂	2¹/₂	0

Nutrients Per Day

Calories: 1,993	**Carbohydrate:** 283 g
Total fat: 64 g	**Protein:** 93 g
Calories from fat: 29%	**Calcium:** 1,616 mg
Saturated fat: 13 g	**Magnesium:** 537 mg
Calories from saturated fat: 6%	**Potassium:** 4,693 mg
Cholesterol: 71 mg	**Fiber:** 32 g
Sodium: 2,069 mg	

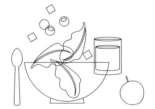

*recipe on page 199

My Shopping List

Make a shopping list. Include the items you need for your menus and any low-calorie basics you need to restock in your kitchen.

Dairy Case

- ☐ Fat-free (skim) or low-fat (1%) milk
- ☐ Low-fat or reduced fat cottage cheese
- ☐ Fat-free cottage cheese
- ☐ Low-fat or reduced fat cheeses
- ☐ Fat-free or low-fat yogurt
- ☐ Light or diet margarine (tub, squeeze, or spray)
- ☐ Fat-free or reduced fat sour cream
- ☐ Fat-free cream cheese
- ☐ Eggs/egg substitute
- ☐ _____

Breads, Muffins, and Rolls

- ☐ Bread, bagels, or pita bread
- ☐ English muffins
- ☐ Yeast breads (whole wheat, rye, pumpernickel, multi-grain, or raisin)
- ☐ Corn tortillas (not fried)
- ☐ Low-fat flour tortillas
- ☐ Fat-free biscuit mix
- ☐ Rice crackers
- ☐ Challah
- ☐ _____

Cereals, Crackers, Rice, Noodles, and Pasta

- ☐ Plain cereal, dry or cooked
- ☐ Saltines, soda crackers (low-sodium or unsalted tops)
- ☐ Graham crackers
- ☐ Other low-fat crackers
- ☐ Rice (brown, white, etc.)
- ☐ Pasta (noodles, spaghetti)
- ☐ Bulgur, couscous, or kasha
- ☐ Potato mixes (made without fat)
- ☐ Wheat mixes
- ☐ Tabouli grain salad

- ☐ Hominy
- ☐ Polenta
- ☐ Polvillo
- ☐ Hominy grits
- ☐ Quinoa
- ☐ Millet
- ☐ Aramanth
- ☐ Oatmeal
- ☐ _____

Meat Case

- ☐ White meat chicken and turkey (skin off)
- ☐ Fish (not battered)
- ☐ Beef, round or sirloin
- ☐ Extra lean ground beef such as ground round
- ☐ Pork tenderloin
- ☐ 95% fat-free lunch meats or low-fat deli meats
- ☐ _____

Meat Equivalents:
- ☐ Tofu (or bean curd)
- ☐ Beans (see bean list)
- ☐ Eggs/egg substitutes (see dairy list)
- ☐ _____

Fruit (fresh, canned, and frozen)

Fresh Fruit:
- ☐ Apples
- ☐ Bananas
- ☐ Peaches
- ☐ Oranges
- ☐ Pears
- ☐ Grapes
- ☐ Grapefruit
- ☐ Apricots
- ☐ Dried Fruits
- ☐ Cherries
- ☐ Plums

- ☐ Melons
- ☐ Lemons
- ☐ Limes
- ☐ Plantains
- ☐ Mangoes
- ☐ _____

Exotic Fresh Fruit:
- ☐ Kiwi
- ☐ Olives
- ☐ Figs
- ☐ Quinces
- ☐ Currants
- ☐ Persimmons
- ☐ Pomegranates
- ☐ Papaya
- ☐ Zapote
- ☐ Guava
- ☐ Starfruit
- ☐ Litchi nuts
- ☐ Winter melons
- ☐ _____

Canned Fruit (in juice or water):
- ☐ Canned pineapple
- ☐ Applesauce
- ☐ Other canned fruits (mixed or plain)
- ☐ _____

Frozen Fruits (without added sugar):
- ☐ Blueberries
- ☐ Raspberries
- ☐ 100% fruit juice
- ☐ _____

Dried Fruit:
- ☐ Raisins/dried fruit (these tend to be higher in calories than fresh fruit)
- ☐ _____

Vegetables (fresh, canned, and frozen)

Fresh Vegetables:
- [ ] Broccoli
- [ ] Peas
- [ ] Corn
- [ ] Cauliflower
- [ ] Squash
- [ ] Green beans
- [ ] Green leafy vegetables
- [ ] Spinach
- [ ] Lettuce
- [ ] Cabbage
- [ ] Artichokes
- [ ] Cucumber
- [ ] Asparagus
- [ ] Mushrooms
- [ ] Carrots or celery
- [ ] Onions
- [ ] Potatoes
- [ ] Tomatoes
- [ ] Green peppers
- [ ] Chilies
- [ ] _____

Canned Vegetables
(low-sodium or no-salt-added):
- [ ] Canned tomatoes
- [ ] Tomato sauce or pasta
- [ ] Other canned vegetables
- [ ] Canned vegetable soup, reduced sodium

Frozen Vegetables:
(without added fats):
- [ ] Broccoli
- [ ] Spinach
- [ ] Mixed medley, etc.
- [ ] _____

Exotic Fresh Vegetables
- [ ] Okra
- [ ] Eggplant
- [ ] Grape leaves
- [ ] Mustard greens
- [ ] Kale
- [ ] Leeks
- [ ] Bamboo shoots
- [ ] Chinese celery
- [ ] Bok choy
- [ ] Napa cabbage
- [ ] Seaweed
- [ ] Rhubarb
- [ ] _____

Beans and Legumes
(if canned, no-salt-added)
- [ ] Lentils
- [ ] Black beans
- [ ] Red beans (kidney beans)
- [ ] Navy beans
- [ ] Black beans
- [ ] Pinto beans
- [ ] Black-eyed peas
- [ ] Fava beans
- [ ] Italian white beans
- [ ] Great white northern beans
- [ ] Chickpeas (garbanzo beans)
- [ ] Dried beans, peas, and lentils (without flavoring packets)
- [ ] _____

Baking Items
- [ ] Flour
- [ ] Sugar
- [ ] Imitation butter (flakes or buds)
- [ ] Non-stick cooking spray
- [ ] Canned evaporated milk— fat-free (skim) or reduced fat (2%)
- [ ] Non-fat dry milk powder
- [ ] Cocoa powder, unsweetened
- [ ] Baking powder
- [ ] Baking soda
- [ ] Cornstarch
- [ ] Unflavored gelatin
- [ ] Gelatin, any flavor (reduced calorie)
- [ ] Pudding mixes (reduced calorie)
- [ ] Angel food cake mix
- [ ] _____

Frozen Foods
- [ ] Fish fillets—unbreaded
- [ ] Egg substitute
- [ ] 100 percent fruit juices (no-sugar-added)
- [ ] Fruits (no-sugar-added)
- [ ] Vegetables (plain)
- [ ] _____

Condiments, Sauces, Seasonings, and Spreads
- [ ] Fat-free or low-fat salad dressings
- [ ] Mustard (Dijon, etc.)
- [ ] Catsup
- [ ] Barbecue sauce
- [ ] Jam, jelly, or honey
- [ ] Spices
- [ ] Flavored vinegars
- [ ] Hoisin sauce and plum sauce
- [ ] Salsa or picante sauce
- [ ] Canned green chilies
- [ ] Soy sauce (low-sodium)
- [ ] Bouillon cubes/granules (low-sodium)
- [ ] _____

Beverages
- [ ] No-calorie drink mixes
- [ ] Reduced calorie juices
- [ ] Unsweetened iced tea
- [ ] Carbonated water
- [ ] Water
- [ ] _____

Nuts and Seeds
- [ ] Almonds, unsalted
- [ ] Mixed nuts, unsalted
- [ ] Peanuts, unsalted
- [ ] Walnuts
- [ ] Sesame seeds
- [ ] Pumpkin seeds, unsalted
- [ ] Sunflower seeds, unsalted
- [ ] Cashews, unsalted
- [ ] Pecans, unsalted
- [ ] _____

Fats and Oils
- [ ] Soft (tub) margarine
- [ ] Mayonnaise, low-fat
- [ ] Canola oil
- [ ] Corn oil
- [ ] Olive oil
- [ ] Safflower oil
- [ ] _____

Tips for Healthy Substitutes

These lower-calorie alternatives provide new ideas for old favorites. When making a food choice, remember to consider vitamins and minerals. Some foods provide most of their calories from sugar and fat but give you few, if any, vitamins and minerals.

This guide is not meant to be an exhaustive list. We stress reading labels to find out just how many calories are in the specific products you decide to buy.

If you usually buy:	Try these:
Milk and Milk Products	
☐ Evaporated whole milk	☐ Evaporated fat-free (skim) or reduced fat (2%) milk
☐ Whole milk	☐ Fat-free (skim), low-fat (1%), or reduced fat (2%) milk
☐ Ice cream	☐ Sorbet and ices, sherbet, and low-fat or fat-free frozen yogurt
☐ Whipping cream	☐ Imitation whipped cream (made with fat-free [skim] milk)
☐ Sour cream	☐ Plain low-fat yogurt
☐ Cream cheese	☐ Neufchatel or "light" cream cheese or fat-free cream cheese
☐ Cheese (cheddar, Swiss, or jack)	☐ Reduced calorie cheese, low-calorie processed cheeses, etc.
☐ American cheese	☐ Fat-free cheese
	☐ Fat-free American cheese or other types of fat-free cheeses
☐ Regular (4%) cottage cheese	☐ Low-fat (1%) or reduced fat (2%) cottage cheese
☐ Whole milk mozzarella cheese	☐ Part-skim milk, low-moisture mozzarella cheese
☐ Whole milk ricotta cheese	☐ Part-skim milk ricotta cheese
☐ Coffee cream (1/2 and 1/2) or non-dairy creamer (liquid or powder)	☐ Low-fat (1%) or reduced fat (2%) milk or non-fat dry milk powder
Cereals, Grains, and Pastas	
☐ Ramen noodles	☐ Rice or noodles (spaghetti, macaroni, etc.)
☐ Pasta with white sauce (Alfredo)	☐ Pasta with red sauce (marinara)
☐ Pasta with cheese sauce	☐ Pasta with vegetables (primavera)
☐ Granola	☐ Bran flakes, crispy rice, etc.
	☐ Cooked grits or oatmeal
	☐ Reduced-fat granola
☐ White rice	☐ Brown rice
Meats, Fish, and Poultry	
☐ Cold cuts or lunch meats (bologna, salami, liverwurst, etc.)	☐ Low-fat cold cuts (95% to 97% fat-free lunch meats or low-fat pressed meats)
☐ Hot dogs (regular)	☐ Lower-fat hot dogs
☐ Bacon or sausage	☐ Canadian bacon or lean ham
☐ Regular ground beef	☐ Extra lean ground beef such as ground round or ground turkey (read labels)

If you usually buy:	Try these:
Meats, Fish, and Poultry (continued)	
☐ Chicken or turkey with skin, duck, or goose	☐ Chicken or turkey without skin (white meat)
☐ Oil-packed tuna	☐ Water-packed tuna (rinse to reduce sodium content)
☐ Beef (chuck, rib, or brisket)	☐ Beef (round or loin) (trimmed of external fat) (choose select grades)
☐ Pork (spareribs or untrimmed loin)	☐ Pork tenderloin or trimmed, lean smoked ham
☐ Frozen breaded fish or fried fish (homemade or commercial)	☐ Fish or shellfish, unbreaded (fresh, frozen, or canned in water)
☐ Whole eggs	☐ Egg whites or egg substitutes
☐ Frozen TV dinners (containing more than 13 grams of fat per serving)	☐ Frozen TV dinners (containing less than 13 grams of fat per serving and lower in sodium)
☐ Chorizo sausage	☐ Turkey sausage, drained well (read label)
	☐ Vegetarian sausage (made with tofu)
Baked Goods	
☐ Croissants, brioches, etc.	☐ Hard french rolls or soft brown 'n serve rolls
☐ Donuts, sweet rolls, muffins, scones, or pastries	☐ English muffins, bagels, reduced fat or fat-free muffins or scones
☐ Party crackers	☐ Low-fat crackers (choose lower in sodium)
	☐ Saltine or soda crackers (choose lower in sodium)
☐ Cake (pound, chocolate or yellow)	☐ Cake (angel food, white, or gingerbread)
☐ Cookies	☐ Fat-free or reduced fat cookies (graham crackers, ginger snaps, or fig bars) (compare calorie level)
Snacks and Sweets	
☐ Nuts	☐ Popcorn (air-popped or light microwave), fruits, vegetables
☐ Ice cream, for example, cones or bars	☐ Frozen yogurt, frozen fruit, or chocolate pudding bars
☐ Custards or puddings (made with whole milk)	☐ Puddings (made with fat-free milk)
Fats, Oils, and Salad Dressings	
☐ Regular margarine or butter	☐ Light spread margarines, diet margarine, or whipped butter, tub or squeeze bottle
☐ Regular mayonaise	☐ Light or diet mayonnaise or mustard
☐ Regular salad dressings	☐ Fat-free or reduced calorie salad dressings, lemon juice, or plain, herb-flavored, or wine vinegar
☐ Butter or margarine on toast or bread	☐ Jelly, jam, or honey on bread or toast
	☐ Non-stick cooking spray for stir-frying or sautéing
☐ Oils, shortening, or lard	☐ As a substitute for oil or butter, use applesauce or prune purée in baked goods
Miscellaneous	
☐ Canned cream soups	☐ Canned broth-based soups (low-sodium)
☐ Gravy (homemade with fat and/or milk)	☐ Gravy mixes made with water or homemade with the fat skimmed off and fat-free milk
☐ Fudge sauce	☐ Chocolate syrup
☐ Guacamole dip or refried beans with lard	☐ Salsa

Tips for Using the Food Label

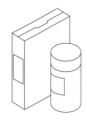

Most packaged foods have a Nutrition Facts label. Here are some tips for reading the label and making smart food choices:

Check servings and calories. Look at the serving size and how many servings you are actually eating.

> **tip:** If you eat 2 servings of a food, you will consume double the calories and double the % Daily Value (% DV) of the nutrients listed on the Nutrition Facts label.

Make your calories count. Look at the calories on the label and compare them with the nutrients they offer.

> **tip:** When you look at a food's nutrition label, first check the calories, and then check the nutrients to decide whether the food is worth eating.

Eat less sugar. Foods with added sugars may provide calories, but few essential nutrients. So, look for foods and beverages low in added sugars. Read the ingredient list, and make sure added sugars are not one of the first few ingredients.

> **tip:** Names for added sugars (caloric sweeteners) include sucrose, glucose, high fructose corn syrup, corn syrup, maple syrup, and fructose.

Know your fats. Look for foods low in saturated and *trans* fats, and cholesterol, to help reduce the risk of heart disease. Most of the fats you eat should be polyunsaturated and monounsaturated fats, such as those in fish, nuts, and vegetable oils.

> **tip:** Fat should be in the range of 20% to 35% of the calories you eat.

Reduce sodium (salt); increase potassium. Research shows that eating less than 2,300 milligrams of sodium (about 1 tsp of salt) per day may reduce the risk of high blood pressure. Older adults tend to be salt-sensitive. If you are older adult or salt-sensitive, aim to eat no more than 1,500 milligrams of sodium each day—the equivalent of about 3/4 teaspoon. To meet the daily potassium recommendation of at least 4,700 milligrams, consume fruits and vegetables, and fat-free and low-fat milk products that are sources of potassium including: sweet potatoes, beet greens, white potatoes, white beans, plain yogurt, prune juice, and bananas. These counteract some of sodium's effects on blood pressure.

> **tip:** Most sodium you eat is likely to come from processed foods, not from the salt shaker. Read the Nutrition Facts label, and choose foods lower in sodium and higher in potassium.

Use the % Daily Value (% DV) column: 5% DV or less is low, and 20% DV or more is high.

Keep these low: saturated and *trans* fats, cholesterol, and sodium.

Get enough of these: potassium and fiber, vitamins A, C, and D, calcium, and iron.

Check the calories: 400 or more calories per serving of a single food item is high.

Nutrition Facts

Serving Size 1 cup (228g)
Servings Per Container 2

Start here

Amount Per Serving

Check calories

Calories 250   Calories from Fat 110

                              % Daily Value*

Quick guide to % DV

Total Fat 12g	**18%**
Saturated Fat 3g	**15%**
Trans Fat 3g	

5% or less is low
20% or more is high

Cholesterol 30mg	**10%**
Sodium 470mg	**20%**

Limit these

Potassium 700mg	**20%**
Total Carbohydrate 31g	**10%**

Get enough of these

Dietary Fiber 0g	0%
Sugars 5g	
Protein 5g	

Vitamin A	**4%**
Vitamin C	**2%**
Calcium	**20%**
Iron	**4%**

Footnote

* Percent Daily Values are based on a 2,000 calorie diet. Your Daily Values may be higher or lower depending on your calorie needs.

	Calories:	2,000	2,500
Total Fat	Less than	65g	80g
Sat Fat	Less than	20g	25g
Cholesterol	Less than	300mg	300mg
Sodium	Less than	2,400mg	2,400mg
Total Carbohydrate		300g	375g
Dietary Fiber		25g	30g

My Physical Activity Tracker

For the week of _____

My goal for this week is:	Cardio or Aerobic 30 minutes most days of the week	Strength Training at least 2 days a week
Monday Notes to myself:	☐ Today's Goal My Activities:	☐ Today's Goal My Activities:
Tuesday Notes to myself:	☐ Today's Goal My Activities:	☐ Today's Goal My Activities:
Wednesday Notes to myself:	☐ Today's Goal My Activities:	☐ Today's Goal My Activities:
Thursday Notes to myself:	☐ Today's Goal My Activities:	☐ Today's Goal My Activities:
Friday Notes to myself:	☐ Today's Goal My Activities:	☐ Today's Goal My Activities:
Saturday Notes to myself:	☐ Today's Goal My Activities:	☐ Today's Goal My Activities:
Sunday Notes to myself:	☐ Today's Goal My Activities:	☐ Today's Goal My Activities:

Cardio or Aerobic: Moderate Physical Activity—You feel your heart beat faster and you breathe faster too. Vigorous Physical Activity—You have a large increase in breathing and heart rate. Conversation is difficult or "broken."

Strength Training: Sometimes called resistance exercises—You work your muscles against resistance using weights or gravity (for example, push-ups). Try 6-8 strength-training exercises of 8-12 repetitions of each exercise.

To track your physical activity online, visit www.presidentschallenge.org.

My Physical Activity Tracker

For the week of _____

My goal for this week is:	Cardio or Aerobic	Strength Training
	30 minutes most days of the week	at least 2 days a week
Monday Notes to myself:	☐ Today's Goal My Activities:	☐ Today's Goal My Activities:
Tuesday Notes to myself:	☐ Today's Goal My Activities:	☐ Today's Goal My Activities:
Wednesday Notes to myself:	☐ Today's Goal My Activities:	☐ Today's Goal My Activities:
Thursday Notes to myself:	☐ Today's Goal My Activities:	☐ Today's Goal My Activities:
Friday Notes to myself:	☐ Today's Goal My Activities:	☐ Today's Goal My Activities:
Saturday Notes to myself:	☐ Today's Goal My Activities:	☐ Today's Goal My Activities:
Sunday Notes to myself:	☐ Today's Goal My Activities:	☐ Today's Goal My Activities:

Cardio or Aerobic: Moderate Physical Activity—You feel your heart beat faster and you breathe faster too. Vigorous Physical Activity—You have a large increase in breathing and heart rate. Conversation is difficult or "broken."

Strength Training: Sometimes called resistance exercises—You work your muscles against resistance using weights or gravity (for example, push-ups). Try 6-8 strength-training exercises of 8-12 repetitions of each exercise.

To track your physical activity online, visit www.presidentschallenge.org.

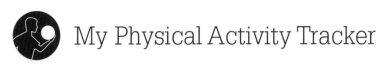

My Physical Activity Tracker

For the week of _____

My goal for this week is:	Cardio or Aerobic	Strength Training
	30 minutes most days of the week	at least 2 days a week
Monday Notes to myself:	☐ Today's Goal My Activities:	☐ Today's Goal My Activities:
Tuesday Notes to myself:	☐ Today's Goal My Activities:	☐ Today's Goal My Activities:
Wednesday Notes to myself:	☐ Today's Goal My Activities:	☐ Today's Goal My Activities:
Thursday Notes to myself:	☐ Today's Goal My Activities:	☐ Today's Goal My Activities:
Friday Notes to myself:	☐ Today's Goal My Activities:	☐ Today's Goal My Activities:
Saturday Notes to myself:	☐ Today's Goal My Activities:	☐ Today's Goal My Activities:
Sunday Notes to myself:	☐ Today's Goal My Activities:	☐ Today's Goal My Activities:

Cardio or Aerobic: Moderate Physical Activity—You feel your heart beat faster and you breathe faster too. Vigorous Physical Activity—You have a large increase in breathing and heart rate. Conversation is difficult or "broken."

Strength Training: Sometimes called resistance exercises—You work your muscles against resistance using weights or gravity (for example, push-ups). Try 6-8 strength-training exercises of 8-12 repetitions of each exercise.

To track your physical activity online, visit www.presidentschallenge.org.

My Physical Activity Tracker

For the week of _____

My goal for this week is:	Cardio or Aerobic	Strength Training
	30 minutes most days of the week	at least 2 days a week
Monday Notes to myself:	☐ Today's Goal My Activities:	☐ Today's Goal My Activities:
Tuesday Notes to myself:	☐ Today's Goal My Activities:	☐ Today's Goal My Activities:
Wednesday Notes to myself:	☐ Today's Goal My Activities:	☐ Today's Goal My Activities:
Thursday Notes to myself:	☐ Today's Goal My Activities:	☐ Today's Goal My Activities:
Friday Notes to myself:	☐ Today's Goal My Activities:	☐ Today's Goal My Activities:
Saturday Notes to myself:	☐ Today's Goal My Activities:	☐ Today's Goal My Activities:
Sunday Notes to myself:	☐ Today's Goal My Activities:	☐ Today's Goal My Activities:

Cardio or Aerobic: Moderate Physical Activity—You feel your heart beat faster and you breathe faster too. Vigorous Physical Activity—You have a large increase in breathing and heart rate. Conversation is difficult or "broken."

Strength Training: Sometimes called resistance exercises—You work your muscles against resistance using weights or gravity (for example, push-ups). Try 6-8 strength-training exercises of 8-12 repetitions of each exercise.

To track your physical activity online, visit www.presidentschallenge.org.

My Physical Activity Tracker

For the week of _____

My goal for this week is:	Cardio or Aerobic	Strength Training
	30 minutes most days of the week	at least 2 days a week
Monday Notes to myself:	☐ Today's Goal My Activities:	☐ Today's Goal My Activities:
Tuesday Notes to myself:	☐ Today's Goal My Activities:	☐ Today's Goal My Activities:
Wednesday Notes to myself:	☐ Today's Goal My Activities:	☐ Today's Goal My Activities:
Thursday Notes to myself:	☐ Today's Goal My Activities:	☐ Today's Goal My Activities:
Friday Notes to myself:	☐ Today's Goal My Activities:	☐ Today's Goal My Activities:
Saturday Notes to myself:	☐ Today's Goal My Activities:	☐ Today's Goal My Activities:
Sunday Notes to myself:	☐ Today's Goal My Activities:	☐ Today's Goal My Activities:

Cardio or Aerobic: Moderate Physical Activity—You feel your heart beat faster and you breathe faster too. Vigorous Physical Activity—You have a large increase in breathing and heart rate. Conversation is difficult or "broken."

Strength Training: Sometimes called resistance exercises—You work your muscles against resistance using weights or gravity (for example, push-ups). Try 6-8 strength-training exercises of 8-12 repetitions of each exercise.

To track your physical activity online, visit www.presidentschallenge.org.

Part IV

Recipes and Resources

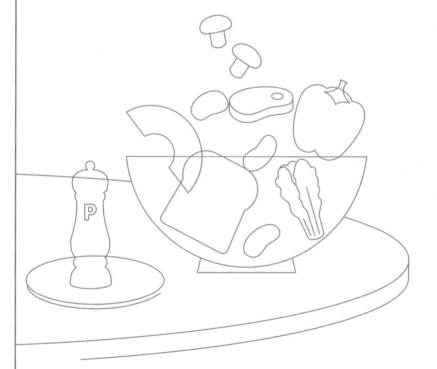

Introduction

An essential part of becoming a Healthier You is making healthy choices. This part of the book will give you some of the tools to stay on track. One of the simplest and most effective healthy choices you can make is to know what you are eating. Cooking at home is one sure-fire way to plan and keep track of calories, portion sizes, nutrients, and all of that other good stuff. Unfortunately, many people avoid cooking at home either because they feel that their cooking skills aren't up to par, don't have the time, or prefer the taste and quality of meals eaten out. This doesn't have to be the case! If you are one of those people, don't worry—we can help!

Here are almost 100 easy-to-make, fun, and delicious recipes. They are "heart healthy." We know that because they were developed by researchers and nutritionists with the HHS National Institutes of Health. No advanced cooking skills required, and they taste great.

The recipes are for appetizers, soups, breads, beef, poultry, fish, vegetables, pasta, rice, sauces, desserts, great vegetarian dishes, and more! On the next page, they are categorized by the amount of time they take to prepare AND cook—from start to finish, all less than 90 minutes total. Since many of us want to save money by preparing our own meals, we've provided some healthy recipes that will be satisfying for the cost-conscious. If you have children that want to help make healthy meals, we have kid-friendly recipes as well.

There are multi-cultural dishes for a variety of tastes, and the best part is that each one is healthy. And you will know that because nutrition information is provided for each recipe. This information includes calories, total fat, saturated fat, cholesterol, and sodium for all recipes. Since you can see the ingredients, you know EXACTLY what is in each serving you eat—a great advantage to cooking your own food—nothing is HIDDEN. We hope you will enjoy the recipes and experiment a little! Make them your own. But be aware of what ingredients you are adding in the process (that means no adding saturated fat and salt!).

Becoming a Healthier You doesn't stop here! Check out the list of government Web resources that you can use to access up-to-date information, advice, and tips for maintaining your progress. You'll find resources for just about every aspect of being healthy. Plus, there are resources for kids (including some really cool teen and tween sites) and older Americans. You'll also find: cultural-specific suggestions, physical activity ideas, nutritional information, menu planning, and shopping tips. There is even a resource for finding recreation areas and parks near you to get out there, be active, and enjoy the scenery!

We also have some great cost-savings tips, tips for using spices to add new flavor and use less salt, food shopping lists, and information on keeping food safe—all tools that will keep you being a Healthier You.

Recipes

*   Kid-friendly
**   Need to marinate
*** Need to soak beans overnight

≤ 30 mins

Toppings/Sauces/Dressings
Chili and Spice Seasoning
Fresh Salsa
Hot 'N Spicy Seasoning
Vinaigrette Salad Dressing
Yogurt Salad Dressing

Breakfast
Applesauce Pancakes
Cinnamon-Sprinkled French Toast*
Fruity Granola Yogurt Parfait*
Huevos Con Turkey Sausage*
Oven-Baked Pancakes
    Whole Wheat Pancakes
    Three-Grain Pancakes
Springtime Cereal

Appetizers/Soups/Salads
Cannery Row Soup
Chicken Salad
Corn Chowder
Gazpacho
Spinach Salad for Spring and Summer
Sunshine Salad
Tuna Salad
Waldorf Salad

Entrées
BEEF:
Beef Stroganoff
Perky Picadillo
Southwest Salad
Stir-Fried Beef and Chinese Vegetables
Stir-Fried Beef and Potatoes

LAMB:
Shish Kabob

CHICKEN:
20-Minute Chicken Creole
Baked Chicken Nuggets
Chicken Marsala
Chicken Oriental
Chicken and Vegetables

TURKEY:
Turkey Patties
Turkey Stir-Fry

FISH:
Baked Salmon Dijon
Baked Trout Olé
Scallop Kabobs
Spicy Baked Fish

VEGETARIAN:
Frittata Primavera

≤ 30 mins (continued)

Sides
Brown or White Rice
Caribbean Pink Beans***
Green Beans Sauté
Oriental Rice
Scallion Rice
Sunshine Rice
Vegetables with a Touch of Lemon

Desserts
Mousse à la Banana
Rainbow Fruit Salad

≤ 60 mins

Breads
Carrot Raisin Bread
Good-for-You Cornbread
Homestyle Biscuits

Appetizers/Soups/Salads
Bean and Macaroni Soup
Mexican Pozole
Minestrone Soup
Pupusas Revueltas with Chicken

Entrées
BEEF:
Beef Casserole
Black Skillet Beef with Greens
    and Red Potatoes

CHICKEN:
Barbecued Chicken
Chicken Ratatouille
Chicken and Spanish Rice
Chicken Stew
Grilled Chicken with Green Chile Sauce**

Entrées (continued)
TURKEY:
Spaghetti with Turkey Meat Sauce
Turkey Meatloaf
Turkey Stuffed Cabbage

FISH:
Catfish Stew and Rice
Mediterranean Baked Fish
Mouth-Watering Oven-Fried Fish

VEGETARIAN:
Classic Macaroni and Cheese
Parmesan Rice and Pasta Pilaf
Summer Vegetable Spaghetti
Vegetarian Spaghetti Sauce

Sides
New Orleans Red Beans
New Potato Salad
Smothered Greens with Turkey

≤ 60 mins (continued)

Desserts
1-2-3 Peach Cobbler
Baked Apple Slices
Oatmeal Cookies
Peach Cake
Peach-Apple Crisp
Rice Pudding
Sweet Potato Custard
Winter Crisp
   Summer Crisp

≤ 90 mins

Breakfast
Zucchini Breakfast Bread

Breads
Banana-Nut Bread

Entrées
CHICKEN:
Chicken and Rice
Spicy Southern Barbecued Chicken**
Yosemite Chicken Stew and Dumplings

VEGETARIAN:
Italian Vegetable Bake
Vegetable Stew
Zucchini Lasagna

Sides
Wonderful Stuffed Potatoes

Desserts
Apple Coffee Cake
Frosted Cake

≤ 30 mins   Toppings/Sauces/Dressings

Chili and Spice Seasoning

This spicy seasoning will heat up your catfish stew—and other dishes too.

$1/4$ cup paprika
2 Tbsp dried oregano, crushed
2 tsp chili powder
1 tsp garlic powder
1 tsp black pepper
$1/2$ tsp red (cayenne) pepper
$1/2$ tsp dry mustard

1. Mix together all ingredients. Store in airtight container.

Yield: $1/3$ cup
Serving size: 1 Tbsp

Each serving provides:
Calories: 26
Total fat: 1 g
Saturated fat: 0 g

Cholesterol: 0 mg
Sodium: 13 mg
Fiber: 2 g
Protein: 1 g
Carbohydrate: 5 g
Potassium: 180 mg

≤ 30 mins   Toppings/Sauces/Dressings

Fresh Salsa

Fresh herbs add flavor—so you can use less salt.

6 tomatoes, preferably Roma (or 3 large tomatoes)
$^1/_2$ medium onion, finely chopped
1 clove garlic, finely minced
2 serrano or jalapeno peppers, finely chopped
3 Tbsp cilantro, chopped
$^1/_8$ tsp oregano, finely crushed
$^1/_8$ tsp salt
$^1/_8$ tsp pepper
$^1/_2$ avocado, diced (black skin)
juice of 1 lime

1. Combine all ingredients in a glass bowl.
2. Serve immediately or refrigerate and serve within 4 or 5 hours.

Yield: 8 servings
Serving size: $^1/_2$ cup

Each serving provides:
Calories: 42
Total fat: 2 g
Saturated fat: Less than 1 g
Cholesterol: 0 mg

Sodium: 44 mg
Calcium: 12 mg
Iron: 1 mg
Fiber: 2 g
Protein: 1 g
Carbohydrate: 7 g
Potassium: 337 mg

≤ 30 mins   **Toppings/Sauces/Dressings**

Hot 'N Spicy Seasoning

Serving tip: Try this mix with meat, poultry, fish, or vegetable dishes. Use it instead of salt—even in the salt shaker.

1¹/₂ tsp white pepper
¹/₂ tsp cayenne pepper
¹/₂ tsp black pepper
1 tsp onion powder
1¹/₄ tsp garlic powder
1 Tbsp basil, dried
1¹/₂ tsp thyme, dried

1. Mix all ingredients together. Store in an airtight container.

Yield: ¹/₃ cup
Serving size: ¹/₂ tsp

Each serving provides:
Calories: 1
Total fat: 1 g
Saturated fat: 0 g
Cholesterol: 0 mg

Sodium: 0 mg
Fiber: 0 g
Protein: 0 g
Carbohydrate: less than 1 g
Potassium: 4 mg

Vinaigrette Salad Dressing

1 bulb garlic, separated and peeled
1/2 cup water
1 Tbsp red wine vinegar
1/4 tsp honey
1 Tbsp virgin olive oil
1/4 tsp black pepper

1. Place the garlic cloves into a small saucepan and pour enough water (about 1/2 cup) to cover them.
2. Bring water to a boil, then reduce heat and simmer until garlic is tender, about 15 minutes.
3. Reduce the liquid to 2 tablespoons and increase the heat for 3 minutes.
4. Pour the contents into a small sieve over a bowl, and with a wooden spoon, mash the garlic through the sieve into the bowl.
5. Whisk the vinegar into the garlic mixture; incorporate the oil and seasoning.

Yield: 4 servings
Serving size: 2 Tbsp

Each serving provides:
Calories: 32
Total fat: 3 g
Saturated fat: less than 1 g

Cholesterol: 0 mg
Sodium: 0 mg
Fiber: 0 g
Protein: 0 g
Carbohydrate: 1 g
Potassium: 6 mg

Yogurt Salad Dressing

8 oz plain yogurt, fat-free
1/4 cup mayonnaise, low-fat
2 Tbsp chives, dried
2 Tbsp dill, dried
2 Tbsp lemon juice

1. Mix all ingredients in bowl and refrigerate.

Yield: 8 servings
Serving size: 2 Tbsp

Each serving provides:
Calories: 39
Total fat: 2 g
Saturated fat: less than 0 g
Cholesterol: 3 mg

Sodium: 66 mg
Fiber: 0 g
Protein: 2 g
Carbohydrate: 4 g
Potassium: 110 mg
Calcium: 76 mg
Magnesium: 10 mg

≤ 30 mins   **Breakfast**

Applesauce Pancakes

1¹/₄ cups milk, low-fat
2 large fresh eggs, beaten or
¹/₂ cup whole frozen eggs (4), thawed
¹/₄ cup vegetable oil (2 Tbsp)
2 cups canned applesauce (1 lb 2 oz)
3 cups all-purpose flour (15 oz)
2 Tbsp baking powder
1 tsp salt
¹/₄ cup sugar
¹/₄ tsp ground cinnamon

1. In a mixing bowl, use the paddle attachment on low speed to combine milk, eggs, oil, and applesauce. Mix for 1 minute until blended.
2. Sift in flour, baking powder, salt, sugar, and cinnamon. Using the whip attachment on low speed, mix batter for 15 seconds until combined. Scrape down the sides of the bowl. Increase speed to medium and mix for 1 minute.
3. Portion batter with level No. 20 scoop (3¹/₃ Tbsp) onto griddle, which has been heated to 375° F. (If desired, lightly oil griddle surface.)
4. Cook until surface of pancake is covered with bubbles and bottom side is lightly browned, about 2 minutes. Turn and cook until lightly browned on other side, about 1 minute.

Yield: 25 servings: 3 lb 1 oz
Serving size: 1 piece provides the equivalent of 1 piece of bread

Each serving provides:
Calories: 121
Protein: 3 g
Carbohydrate: 19 g

Total fat: 4 g
Saturated fat: 0.7 g
Cholesterol: 20 mg
Vitamin A: 16 RE/60 IU
Vitamin C: 0 mg
Iron: 1 mg
Calcium: 86 mg
Sodium: 0 mg
Fiber: 1 g

≤ 30 mins   Breakfast

Cinnamon-Sprinkled French Toast

2 large eggs
2 Tbsp milk, fat-free
1/2 tsp ground cinnamon, or to taste
2 slices whole wheat bread
1 tsp soft (tub) margarine
4 tsp light pancake syrup

Kids: Crack two eggs into flat-bottomed bowl. Thoroughly whisk in milk and
cinnamon. Dip bread slices, one at a time, into egg mixture in bowl, wetting both
sides. Re-dip, if necessary, until all the egg mixture is absorbed into the bread.

Adults: Meanwhile, heat large, non-stick skillet over medium heat. Add butter.
Place dipped bread slices in skillet. Cook for 2 1/2-3 minutes per side, or until
both sides are golden brown.

Kids: Drizzle with syrup. Serve when warm.

Yield: 2 servings	**Saturated fat:** 3 g
Serving size: 1 slice	**Cholesterol:** 215 mg
	Fiber: 2 g
Each serving provides:	**Sodium:** 250 mg
Calories: 190	**Vitamin A:** 8%
Carbohydrate: 19 g	**Vitamin C:** 0%
Protein: 10 g	**Calcium:** 8%
Total fat: 8 g	**Iron:** 10%

Fruity Granola Yogurt Parfait

Did you know? Commercially available granola is often toasted with oil and honey, making it high in calories. So, it's important to choose low-fat granola, when available.

1/2 cup granola, low-fat
3/4 cup (6-oz container) vanilla or plain yogurt, low-fat
1/2 cup fresh blueberries, raspberries, or sliced strawberries or bananas
(use frozen fruit if fresh isn't available)

Adults: Measure out all ingredients to be used. Provide stemware or clear drinking glass or bowl.

Kids: Layer ingredients any which way you want in a glass, such as half of granola, yogurt, and fruit, then repeat. Eat with a long spoon.

Yield: 1 serving
Serving size: 1 3/4 cups

Each serving provides:
Calories: 410
Carbohydrate: 76 g
Protein: 15 g
Total fat: 6 g

Saturated fat: 2.5 g
Cholesterol: 10 mg
Fiber: 5 g
Sodium: 180 mg
Vitamin A: 25%
Vitamin C: 20%
Calcium: 35%
Iron: 10%

Huevos Con Turkey Sausage

2 tsp vegetable oil
1 small (or 1/2 large) white onion, chopped
1 large tomato, chopped
1/2 lb turkey sausage (preferably hot Italian), squeezed from the skin
4 large eggs
1/4 tsp salt, or to taste
4 small (6-inch) corn or flour tortillas, warm
1 Tbsp chopped fresh cilantro or parsley (optional)

Adults: Heat oil in large skillet over medium-high heat. Add onion and tomato. Sauté while stirring for 1 minute.

Kids: Toss in the turkey sausage. Stir frequently for 10 minutes while breaking apart sausage as you stir.

Kids and Adults: Add eggs and stir (scramble) for 1 additional minute, or until eggs are fully cooked. Sprinkle with salt.

Kids: Serve about 2/3-cup scoop of the Huevos Con Turkey Sausage on top of each corn tortilla.

Yield: 4 servings

Serving size:
1 topped tortilla

Each serving provides:
Calories: 280
Carbohydrate: 19 g
Protein: 17 g
Total fat: 15 g

Saturated fat: 4 g
Cholesterol: 260 mg
Fiber: 2 g
Sodium: 590 mg
Vitamin A: 15%
Vitamin C: 15%
Calcium: 6%
Iron: 10%

Oven-Baked Pancakes

Special tip: For best results, after pouring the batter in the pan, spray the top with vegetable oil to obtain a golden brown color.

3 cups all-purpose flour (15 oz)
2 Tbsp baking powder
1/4 cup sugar
2 tsp salt
2 large fresh eggs or
1/2 cup whole frozen eggs (4), thawed
1/4 cup vegetable oil
3 cups milk, low-fat

1. In a mixing bowl, use the whip attachment on low speed to combine all ingredients for 30 seconds. Scrape the sides of the bowl and mix on medium speed for 1 minute, until batter is smooth.
2. Pour 1 quart 1 cup (2 lb 15 oz) of batter into each lightly greased half-sheet pan (18 inches by 13 inches by 1 inch).
3. To Bake:
   Conventional Oven: 450° F, 10 minutes
   Convection Oven: 400° F,
   8 minutes
   Bake until golden brown.
4. Cut each pan into 25 pieces (5 inches by 5 inches).

Yield: 25 servings: 2 lb 9 oz
Serving size: 1 piece provides the equivalent of 1 slice of bread

Each serving provides:
Calories: 110
Protein: 3 g
Carbohydrate: 17 g

Total fat: 3.1 g
Saturated fat: 0.7 g
Cholesterol: 20 mg
Vitamin A: 26 RE/89 IU
Vitamin C: 0 mg
Iron: 1 mg
Calcium: 106 mg
Sodium: 324 mg
Fiber: 0 g

Variations of Oven-Baked Pancakes

Whole Wheat Pancakes

In Step 1, instead of using 15 oz of all-purpose flour, substitute a mixture of 7 oz (1½ cups) of whole wheat flour and 7 oz (1½ cups) of all-purpose flour. Continue with Steps 1, 2, 3, and 4 as directed.

Three-Grain Pancakes

In Step 1, in place of all-purpose flour, substitute a mixture of 5 oz (1 cup) buckwheat flour, 5 oz (1 cup) enriched bran flour, and 5 oz (1 cup) whole wheat flour. Continue with Steps 1, 2, 3, and 4 as directed.

≤ 30 mins   Breakfast

Springtime Cereal

This recipe provides 1.5 fruit and vegetable servings per person.

³/₄ cup wheat and barley nugget cereal
¹/₄ cup 100% bran cereal
2 tsp toasted sunflower seeds
2 tsp toasted almonds, sliced
1 Tbsp raisins
¹/₂ cup bananas, sliced
1 cup strawberries, sliced
1 cup raspberry or strawberry yogurt, low-fat

1. Mix the wheat and barley nugget cereal, bran cereal, sunflower seeds, and almonds in a medium bowl. Add the raisins, the bananas, and halve the strawberries. Gently stir in the yogurt and divide between two bowls. Scatter the remaining strawberries over the top and enjoy!

Serves: 2 people
Nutrition:
Per serving with low-fat
yogurt: 352 calories
Fat: 6 g
Saturated fat: 1 g
Carbohydrate: 69 g
Sodium: 272 mg
Fiber: 8 g

Per serving with light
yogurt (sugar substitute):
268 calories
Fat: 5 g
Saturated fat: 0 g
Carbohydrate: 53 g
Sodium: 263 mg
Fiber: 9 g

≤ 90 mins   Breakfast

Zucchini Breakfast Bread

Did you know? If you don't have 3 cups of self-rising flour, you can use 3 cups of all-purpose flour + 4 teaspoons baking powder + $1/4$ teaspoon salt.

3 large eggs, beaten
$1^3/4$ cups sugar
$1/2$ cup vegetable oil
$1/2$ cup cinnamon applesauce
1 Tbsp vanilla extract
2 cups zucchini, shredded or grated
3 cups self-rising flour
$1/2$ cup walnuts or pecans, chopped

Adults: Preheat the oven to 350° F.

Kids: Spray a non-stick 9- by 5-inch loaf pan with cooking spray.

Adults: In a large bowl, whisk together the beaten eggs, sugar, oil, applesauce, and vanilla.

Kids: Dump in the zucchini. Stir with a large spoon. Sprinkle in flour. Stir well.

Kids and Adults: Pour batter in the loaf pan. Sprinkle nuts over the batter. Bake for 1 hour, or until a toothpick comes out clean. Cool for 15 minutes on a cooling rack.

Adults: Loosen bread from the sides and remove the bread to cool completely on the rack. Once cool, slice and serve. (Hint: The bread slices even better when partially frozen.) Store individually wrapped leftovers in the freezer.

Yield: 14 servings	**Saturated fat:** 2 g
Serving size: 1 slice	**Cholesterol:** 45 mg
	Fiber: 1 g
Each serving provides:	**Sodium:** 360 mg
Calories: 320	**Vitamin A:** 2%
Carbohydrate: 48 g	**Vitamin C:** 4%
Protein: 5 g	**Calcium:** 10%
Total fat: 12 g	**Iron:** 10%

Carrot Raisin Bread

This tasty bread is low in saturated fat and cholesterol, thanks to the small amount of oil and egg used.

1 1/2 cups all-purpose flour, sifted
1/2 cup sugar
1 tsp baking powder
1/4 tsp baking soda
1/2 tsp salt
1 1/2 tsp ground cinnamon
1/4 tsp ground allspice
1 egg, beaten
1/2 cup water
2 Tbsp vegetable oil
1/2 tsp vanilla
1 1/2 cups carrots, finely shredded
1/4 cup pecans, chopped
1/4 cup golden raisins

1. Preheat oven to 350° F. Lightly oil a 9- by 5- by 3-inch loaf pan.
2. Stir together dry ingredients in large mixing bowl. Make a well in center of dry mixture.
3. In separate bowl, mix together remaining ingredients; add this mixture all at once to dry ingredients. Stir just enough to moisten and evenly distribute carrots.
4. Turn into prepared pan. Bake for 50 minutes or until toothpick inserted in center comes out clean.
5. Cool 5 minutes in pan. Remove from pan and complete cooling on a wire rack before slicing.

Yield: 1 loaf
Serving size: 1/2-inch slice

Each serving provides:
Calories: 99
Total fat: 3 g
Saturated fat: less than 1 g
Cholesterol: 12 mg
Sodium: 97 mg
Fiber: 1 g
Protein: 2 g
Carbohydrate: 17 g
Potassium: 69 mg

≤ 60 mins   Breads

Good-for-You Cornbread

Use 1% buttermilk and a small amount of margarine to make this cornbread lower in saturated fat and cholesterol.

1 cup cornmeal
1 cup flour
1/4 cup white sugar
1 tsp baking powder
1 cup buttermilk, low-fat
1 egg, whole
1/4 cup soft (tub) margarine
1 tsp vegetable oil (to grease baking pan)

1. Preheat oven to 350° F.
2. Mix together cornmeal, flour, sugar, and baking powder.
3. In another bowl, combine buttermilk and egg. Beat lightly.
4. Slowly add buttermilk and egg mixture to the dry ingredients.
5. Add margarine and mix by hand or with a mixer for 1 minute.
6. Bake for 20-25 minutes in an 8- by 8-inch greased baking dish. Cool.
7. Cut into 10 squares.

Yield: 10 servings
Serving size: 1 square

Each serving provides:
Calories: 178
Fat: 6 g
Saturated fat: 1 g

Cholesterol: 22 mg
Sodium: 94 mg
Fiber: 1 g
Protein: 4 g
Carbohydrate: 27 g
Potassium: 132 mg

Homestyle Biscuits

It's easy to make homestyle biscuits with less fat.

2 cups flour
2 tsp baking powder
1/4 tsp baking soda
1/4 tsp salt
2 Tbsp sugar
2/3 cup buttermilk, low-fat
3 Tbsp + 1 tsp vegetable oil

1. Preheat oven to 450° F.
2. In a medium bowl, combine flour, baking powder, baking soda, salt, and sugar.
3. In a small bowl, stir together buttermilk and oil. Pour over flour mixture; stir until well mixed.
4. On a lightly floured surface, knead dough gently for 10-12 strokes.
5. Roll or pat dough to 3/4-inch thickness.
6. Cut with a 2-inch biscuit or cookie cutter, dipping cutter in flour between cuts.
7. Transfer biscuits to an ungreased baking sheet.
8. Bake for 12 minutes or until golden brown. Serve warm.

Yield: 15 servings
Serving size:
1 (2-inch) biscuit

Each serving provides:
Calories: 99
Total fat: 3 g

Saturated fat: less than 1 g
Cholesterol: less than 1 mg
Sodium: 72 mg
Fiber: 1 g
Protein: 2 g
Carbohydrate: 15 g
Potassium: 102 mg

Banana-Nut Bread

Bananas and low-fat buttermilk give this old favorite its moistness and help lower the fat.

1 cup ripe bananas, mashed
1/3 cup buttermilk, low-fat
1/2 cup brown sugar, packed
1/4 cup soft (tub) margarine
1 egg
2 cups all-purpose flour, sifted
1 tsp baking powder
1/2 tsp baking soda
1/2 tsp salt
1/2 cup pecans, chopped

1. Preheat oven to 350° F. Lightly oil two 9- by 5-inch loaf pans.
2. Stir together mashed bananas and buttermilk; set aside.
3. Cream brown sugar and margarine together until light. Beat in egg. Add banana mixture; beat well.
4. Sift together flour, baking powder, baking soda, and salt; add all at once to liquid ingredients. Stir until well blended.
5. Stir in nuts and turn into prepared pan.
6. Bake for 50-55 minutes or until toothpick inserted in center comes out clean. Cool 5 minutes in pan.
7. Remove from pan and complete cooling on a wire rack before slicing.

Yield: 1 loaf	**Cholesterol:** 12 mg
Serving size: 1/2-inch slice	**Sodium:** 138 mg
	Fiber: 1 g
Each serving provides:	**Protein:** 2 g
Calories: 133	**Carbohydrate:** 20 g
Total fat: 5 g	**Potassium:** 114 mg
Saturated fat: 1 g	

Appetizers/Soups/Salads

Cannery Row Soup

Using fish and clam juice makes this tasty soup heart-healthy.

2 lb varied fish fillets (e.g., haddock, perch, flounder, cod, or sole), cut into 1-inch-square cubes
2 Tbsp olive oil
1 clove garlic, minced
3 carrots, cut into thin strips
2 cups celery, sliced
$^1/_2$ cup onion, chopped
$^1/_4$ cup green peppers, chopped
1 can (28 oz) whole tomatoes, cut up, with liquid
1 cup clam juice
$^1/_4$ tsp dried thyme, crushed
$^1/_4$ tsp dried basil, crushed
$^1/_8$ tsp black pepper
$^1/_4$ cup fresh parsley, minced

1. Heat oil in large sauce pan. Sauté garlic, carrots, celery, onion, and green pepper in oil 3 minutes.
2. Add remaining ingredients except parsley and fish. Cover and simmer 10-15 minutes or until vegetables are fork-tender.
3. Add fish and parsley. Simmer, covered, 5-10 minutes more or until fish flakes easily and is opaque. Serve hot.

Yield: 8 servings
Serving size: 1 cup each

Each serving provides:
Calories: 170
Total fat: 5 g
Saturated fat: less than 1 g

Cholesterol: 56 mg
Sodium: 380 mg
Fiber: 3 g
Protein: 22 g
Carbohydrate: 9 g
Potassium: 710 mg

Chicken Salad

Chill out with this simple, yet flavorful dish.

3¹/₄ cups chicken, cooked, cubed, and skinless
¹/₄ cup celery, chopped
1 Tbsp lemon juice
¹/₂ tsp onion powder
¹/₈ tsp salt*
3 Tbsp mayonnaise, low-fat

1. Bake chicken, cut into cubes, and refrigerate.
2. In large bowl, combine rest of ingredients, add chilled chicken and mix well.

Reduce sodium by removing the ¹/₈ tsp of added salt. New sodium content for each serving is 127 mg.

Yield: 5 servings	**Cholesterol:** 77 mg
Serving size: ³/₄ cup	**Sodium:** 179 mg
	Fiber: 0 g
Each serving provides:	**Protein:** 27 g
Calories: 176	**Carbohydrate:** 2 g
Total fat: 6 g	**Potassium:** 236 mg
Saturated fat: 2 g	

≤ 30 mins   Appetizers/Soups/Salads

Corn Chowder

Using low-fat milk instead of cream lowers the saturated fat content in this hearty dish.

1 Tbsp vegetable oil
2 Tbsp celery, finely diced
2 Tbsp onion, finely diced
2 Tbsp green pepper, finely diced
1 package (10 oz) frozen whole kernel corn
1 cup raw potatoes, peeled, diced, and 1/2-inch
2 Tbsp fresh parsley, chopped
1 cup water
1/4 tsp salt
black pepper to taste
1/4 tsp paprika
2 Tbsp flour
2 cups milk, fat-free or low-fat (1%)

1. Heat oil in medium saucepan.
2. Add celery, onion, and green pepper and sauté for 2 minutes.
3. Add corn, potatoes, water, salt, pepper, and paprika. Bring to a boil; reduce heat to medium; and cook, covered, about 10 minutes or until potatoes are tender.
4. Pour 1/2 cup of milk into a jar with tight-fitting lid. Add flour and shake vigorously.
5. Add gradually to cooked vegetables and add remaining milk.
6. Cook, stirring constantly, until mixture comes to a boil and thickens. Serve garnished with chopped fresh parsley.

Yield: 4 servings
Serving size: 1 cup

Each serving provides:
Calories: 186
Total fat: 5 g
Saturated fat: 1 g

Cholesterol: 5 mg
Sodium: 205 mg
Fiber: 4 g
Protein: 7 g
Carbohydrate: 31 g
Potassium: 455 mg

Gazpacho

This classic chilled tomato soup is chock full of garden-fresh vegetables, choles-terol-free, and made with very little added oil.

4 cups tomato juice*
$1/2$ medium onion, peeled and coarsely chopped
1 small green pepper, peeled, cored, seeded, and coarsely chopped
1 small cucumber, peeled, pared, seeded, and coarsely chopped
$1/2$ tsp Worcestershire sauce
1 clove garlic, minced
1 drop hot pepper sauce
$1/8$ tsp cayenne pepper
$1/4$ tsp black pepper
2 Tbsp olive oil
1 large tomato, finely diced
2 Tbsp minced chives or scallion tops
1 lemon, cut into 6 wedges

1. Put 2 cups of tomato juice and all other ingredients except diced tomato, chives, and lemon wedges into the blender.
2. Purée.
3. Slowly add the remaining 2 cups of tomato juice to puréed mixture. Add diced tomato. Chill.
4. Serve icy cold in individual bowls garnished with minced chives and lemon wedges.

Yield: 6 servings
Serving size: 1 cup

Each serving provides:
Calories: 87
Total fat: 5 g

Saturated fat: less than 1 g
Cholesterol: 0 mg
Sodium: 593 mg*

To cut back on sodium, try low-sodium tomato juice.

Spinach Salad for Spring and Summer

This recipe provides 2.5 fruit and vegetable servings per person.

3 cups baby spinach leaves, well washed and dried
1 cup seasonal fresh vegetables or fruits of your choice such as raw sugar snap peas, strawberry halves, blueberries, or peach slices
3 Tbsp vinaigrette salad dressing, low-fat
$1/2$ tsp black pepper

1. Place the spinach and seasonal fruits or vegetables into a large bowl. The more colors you add to your diet, the more nutrients you'll get. Toss with the dressing and serve.

Serves: 2 people

Each serving provides:
(Nutritional information
includes strawberries in
salad):

Calories: 59
Total fat: 2 g
Saturated fat: 0 g
Carbohydrate: 10 g
Sodium: 250 mg
Fiber: 6 g

Sunshine Salad

This recipe provides 2 fruit and vegetable servings per person.

5 cups spinach leaves, packed, washed, and dried well
$1/2$ red onion, sliced thin
$1/2$ red pepper, sliced
1 whole cucumber, sliced
2 oranges, peeled and chopped into bite-size pieces
$1/3$ cup of bottle "lite" vinaigrette dressing (around 15 calories per tablespoon or less)

1. Toss all ingredients together in a large bowl. Add dressing and toss again. Serve immediately.

Serves: 5 people

Each serving provides:
Cholesterol: 0 mg
Fiber: 8 g

Sodium: 200 mg
Calories from Protein: 18%
Calories from Carbohydrate: 62%
Calories from Fat: 20%

Tuna Salad

2 6-oz cans tuna, water pack
$1/2$ cup raw celery, chopped
$1/3$ cup green onions, chopped
$6^1/2$ Tbsp mayonnaise, low-fat

1. Rinse and drain tuna for 5 minutes. Break apart with a fork.
2. Add celery, onion, and mayonnaise and mix well.

Yield: 5 servings
Serving size: $1/2$ cup

Each serving provides:
Calories: 138
Fat: 7 g
Saturated fat: 1 g

Cholesterol: 25 mg
Sodium: 171 mg
Fiber: 0 g
Protein: 16 g
Carbohydrate: 2 g
Potassium: 198 mg

Waldorf Salad

This recipe provides 2.5 fruit and vegetable servings per person.

2 red-skinned crisp apples, try Jongold or Red Delicious (3 cups)
2 Tbsp lemon juice
2 ribs celery, diced (1/2 cup)
2 Tbsp toasted walnuts, chopped
1/4 cup mayonnaise dressing, low-fat
4 cups romaine lettuce, washed and torn into bite-size pieces
1/4 cup raisins

1. Wash and cut the apples into quarters, core, then dice into 3/4-inch pieces. Toss with the lemon juice.
2. Add the celery, walnuts, and mayonnaise dressing. Mix thoroughly.
3. Place the lettuce on four plates or into salad bowls.
4. Scoop the apple mixture onto each salad.
5. Scatter raisins over the top.

Serves: 4 people

Each serving provides:
Calories: 129
Total fat: 4 g

Saturated fat: 0 g
Carbohydrate: 25 g
Sodium: 163 mg
Fiber: 4 g

Bean and Macaroni Soup

This cholesterol-free tasty dish is virtually fat-free and is prepared with only 1 tablespoon of oil for 16 servings.

2 cans (16 oz) great northern beans
1 Tbsp olive oil
1/2 lb fresh mushrooms, sliced
1 cup onion, coarsely chopped
2 cups carrots, sliced
1 cup celery, coarsely chopped
1 clove garlic, minced
3 cups peeled fresh tomatoes, cut up, or
1 1/2 lb canned whole tomatoes, cut up
1 tsp dried sage
1 tsp dried thyme
1/2 tsp dried oregano
black pepper, to taste
1 bay leaf, crumbled
4 cups elbow macaroni, cooked

1. Drain beans and reserve liquid. Rinse beans.
2. Heat oil in a 6-quart kettle; add mushrooms, onion, carrots, celery, and garlic and sauté for 5 minutes.
3. Add tomatoes, sage, thyme, oregano, pepper, and bay leaf.
4. Cover and cook over medium heat 20 minutes. Cook macaroni according to directions on package using unsalted water. Drain when cooked. Do not overcook.
5. Combine reserved bean liquid with water to make 4 cups.
6. Add liquid, beans, and cooked macaroni to vegetable mixture.
7. Bring to a boil; cover and simmer until soup is throughly heated. Stir occasionally.

(continued)

Bean and Macaroni Soup (continued)

Yield: 16 servings

Serving size: 1 cup

Each serving provides:

Calories: 158

Total fat: 1 g

Saturated fat: 1 g

Cholesterol: 0 mg

Sodium: 154 mg*

Fiber: 5 mg

Protein: 8 mg

Carbohydrate: 29 g

Potassium: 524 mg

If canned tomatoes are used, sodium will be higher.

Mexican Pozole

Only a small amount of oil is needed to sauté meat.

2 lb lean beef, cubed
1 Tbsp olive oil
1 large onion, chopped
1 clove garlic, finely chopped
1/4 tsp salt
1/8 tsp pepper
1/4 cup cilantro
1 can (15 oz) stewed tomatoes
2 oz tomato paste
1 can (1 lb 13 oz) hominy

1. In a large pot, heat oil. Sauté beef.
2. Add onion, garlic, salt, pepper, cilantro, and enough water to cover the meat. Cover pot and cook over low heat until meat is tender.
3. Add tomatoes and tomato paste. Continue cooking for about 20 minutes.
4. Add hominy and continue cooking another 15 minutes, stirring occasionally, over low heat. If too thick, add water for desired consistency.

Option: Skinless, boneless chicken breasts may be used instead of beef cubes.

Yield: 10 servings	**Sodium:** 425 mg
Serving size: 1 cup	**Calcium:** 28 mg
	Iron: 3 mg
Each serving provides:	**Fiber:** 4 g
Calories: 253	**Protein:** 22 g
Total fat: 10 g	**Carbohydrate:** 19 g
Saturated fat: 3 g	**Potassium:** 485 mg
Cholesterol: 52 mg	

Minestrone Soup

A cholesterol-free classic Italian vegetable soup brimming with fiber-rich beans, peas, and carrots.

1/4 cup olive oil
1 clove garlic, minced, or 1/8 tsp garlic powder
1 1/3 cups onion, coarsely chopped
1 1/2 cups celery and leaves, coarsely chopped
1 can (6 oz) tomato paste
1 Tbsp fresh parsley, chopped
1 cup sliced carrots, fresh or frozen
4 3/4 cups cabbage, shredded
1 can (1 lb) tomatoes, cut up
1 cup canned red kidney beans, drained and rinsed
1 1/2 cups frozen peas
1 1/2 cups fresh green beans
dash hot sauce
11 cups water
2 cups spaghetti, uncooked and broken

1. Heat oil in a 4-quart saucepan.
2. Add garlic, onion, and celery and sauté about 5 minutes.
3. Add all remaining ingredients except spaghetti, and stir until ingredients are well mixed.
4. Bring to a boil. Reduce heat, cover, and simmer about 45 minutes or until vegetables are tender.
5. Add uncooked spaghetti and simmer 2-3 minutes only.

Yield: 16 servings
Serving size: 1 cup

Each serving provides:
Calories: 112
Total fat: 4 g
Saturated fat: 0 g

Cholesterol: 0 mg
Sodium: 202 mg
Fiber: 4 g
Protein: 4 g
Carbohydrate: 17 g
Potassium: 393 mg

Pupusas Revueltas with Chicken
Ground chicken and low-fat cheese help reduce fat and calories.

1 lb ground chicken breast
1 Tbsp vegetable oil
1/2 lb mozzarella cheese, grated, low-fat
1/2 small onion, finely diced
1 clove garlic, minced
1 medium green pepper, seeded and minced
1 small tomato, finely chopped
1/2 tsp salt
5 cups instant corn flour (masa harina)
6 cups water

1. In a non-stick skillet over low heat, sauté chicken in oil until chicken turns white. Constantly stir the chicken to keep it from sticking.
2. Add onion, garlic, green pepper, and tomato. Cook until chicken mixture is cooked through. Remove skillet from stove and let mixture cool in the refrigerator.
3. While the chicken mixture is cooling, place the flour into a large mixing bowl and stir in enough water to make a stiff tortilla-like dough.
4. When the chicken mixture has cooled, mix in the cheese.
5. Divide the dough into 24 portions. With your hands, roll the dough into balls and flatten each ball into a 1/2-inch-thick circle. Put a spoonful of the chicken mixture into the middle of each circle of dough and bring the edges to the center. Flatten the ball of dough again until it is 1/2-inch thick.
6. In a very hot, iron skillet, cook the pupusas on each side until golden brown.
7. Serve hot with Curtido salvadoreño.

Yield: 12 servings	**Sodium:** 223 mg
Serving size: 2 pupusas	**Calcium:** 149 mg
	Iron: 2 mg
Each serving provides:	**Fiber:** 5 g
Calories: 290	**Protein:** 14 g
Total fat: 7 g	**Carbohydrate:** 38 g
Saturated fat: 3 g	**Potassium:** 272 mg
Cholesterol: 33 mg	

Beef Stroganoff

Using lean top round beef, plain low-fat yogurt, and very little added salt makes this a heart-healthy dish.

1 lb lean beef (top round)
2 tsp vegetable oil
3/4 Tbsp onion, finely chopped
1 lb mushrooms, sliced
1/4 tsp salt
black pepper to taste
1/4 tsp nutmeg
1/2 tsp dried basil
1/4 cup white wine
1 cup plain yogurt, low-fat
6 cups cooked macaroni, cooked in unsalted water

1. Cut beef into 1-inch cubes. Heat 1 teaspoon oil in a non-stick skillet. Sauté onion for 2 minutes.
2. Add beef and sauté for additional 5 minutes. Turn to brown evenly. Remove from pan and keep hot.
3. Add remaining oil to pan; sauté mushrooms.
4. Add beef and onions to pan with seasonings.
5. Add wine and yogurt; gently stir in. Heat, but do not boil.
6. Serve with macaroni.

Note: If thickening is desired, use 2 teaspoons cornstarch; calories are the same as flour, but cornstarch has double thickening power. These calories are not figured into the nutrients per serving.

Yield: 5 servings
Serving size: 6 oz

Each serving provides:
Calories: 499
Total fat: 10 g
Saturated fat: 3 g

Cholesterol: 79 mg
Sodium: 200 mg
Fiber: 4 g
Protein: 41 g
Carbohydrate: 58 g
Potassium: 891 mg

Perky Picadillo

Did you know? You can freeze leftovers of this Cuban dish in an airtight container. When ready to eat, thaw in the refrigerator, then reheat in the microwave until hot (2-3 minutes).

1 Tbsp vegetable oil
1 large yellow onion, chopped
1 large or 2 small green peppers, chopped
3/4 lb lean ground round or sirloin (95% lean)
1 jar (3.5 oz) capers (1/2 cup)
1 tsp garlic salt, or to taste
1/4 tsp black pepper, or to taste
1/2 cup tomato sauce
1/4 cup white grape juice or apple juice

1. Pre-prep all ingredients that need to be chopped.
2. In a large, non-stick skillet, heat the oil over medium-high heat. Sauté the chopped onion and pepper.
3. Add meat and cook for a few minutes while stirring. Add all the remaining ingredients.
4. Reduce heat to medium-low. Let it simmer, uncovered, for 15 minutes while stirring occasionally.
5. Serve the picadillo with rice and beans.

Yield: 6 servings	**Carbohydrate:** 8 g
Serving size: 3/4 cup	**Protein:** 21 g
	Total fat: 10 g
Each serving provides:	**Saturated fat:** 3 g
Calories: 200	**Cholesterol:** 160 mg

Southwest Salad

Note: Garbanzo bean is another name for chickpea.

1/2 cup onions, chopped
1 lb lean ground beef
1 Tbsp chili powder
2 tsp ground cumin
2 tsp oregano
1 cup canned red kidney beans, drained
1 can (15 oz) chickpeas, drained
1 medium tomato, diced
2 cups lettuce
1/2 cup cheddar cheese

1. Cook ground beef and onions in a large skillet until the beef no longer remains pink. Drain.
2. Stir chili powder, oregano, and cumin into beef mixture; cook for 1 minute.
3. Add beans, chickpeas, and tomatoes. Mix gently to combine.
4. Combine lettuce and cheddar cheese in large serving bowl. Portion lettuce and cheese onto four plates. Add 1 cup of beef mixture on top of lettuce and cheese.

Yield: 4 servings
Serving size: about 1/2 cup beef mixture, 1/2 cup lettuce and cheese mixture each

Each serving provides:
Calories: 485
Total fat: 22 g
Saturated fat: 9 g
Cholesterol: 98 mg
Sodium: 411 mg

Stir-Fried Beef and Chinese Vegetables

2 Tbsp dry red wine
1 Tbsp soy sauce
1/2 tsp sugar
1 1/2 tsp gingerroot, peeled and grated
1 lb boneless round steak, fat trimmed and cut across grain into 1 1/2-inch strips
2 Tbsp vegetable oil
2 medium onions, each cut into 8 wedges
1/2 lb fresh mushrooms, rinsed, trimmed, and sliced
2 stalks (1/2 cup) celery, bias cut into 1/4-inch slices
2 small green peppers, cut into thin lengthwise strips
1 cup water chestnuts, drained and sliced
2 Tbsp cornstarch
1/4 cup water

1. Prepare marinade by mixing together wine, soy sauce, sugar, and ginger.
2. Marinate beef in mixture while preparing vegetables.
3. Heat 1 tablespoon of oil in large skillet or wok. Stir-fry onions and mushrooms for 3 minutes over medium-high heat.
4. Add celery and cook for 1 minute. Add remaining vegetables and cook for 2 minutes or until green pepper is tender but crisp. Transfer vegetables to warm bowl.
5. Add remaining 1 tablespoon of oil to skillet. Stir-fry meat in oil for about 2 minutes, or until meat loses its pink color.
6. Blend cornstarch and water. Stir into meat. Cook and stir until thickened. Then return vegetables to skillet. Stir gently and serve.

Yield: 6 servings	**Cholesterol:** 40 mg
Serving size: 6 oz	**Sodium:** 201 mg
	Fiber: 3 g
Each serving provides:	**Protein:** 17 g
Calories: 200	**Carbohydrate:** 12 g
Total fat: 9 g	**Potassium:** 552 mg
Saturated fat: 2 g	

Stir-Fried Beef and Potatoes

Trim fat off beef before cooking.

1¹/₂ lb sirloin steak
2 tsp vegetable oil
1 clove garlic, minced
1 tsp vinegar
¹/₈ tsp salt
¹/₈ tsp pepper
2 large onions, sliced
1 large tomato, sliced
3 cups boiled potatoes, diced

1. Trim fat from steak and cut into small, thin pieces.
2. In a large skillet, heat oil and sauté garlic until garlic is golden. Add steak, vinegar, salt, and pepper.
3. Cook for 6 minutes, stirring beef until brown.
4. Add onion and tomato. Cook until onion is transparent. Serve with boiled potatoes.

Yield: 6 servings	**Saturated fat:** 1 g
Serving size: 1¹/₄ cups	**Cholesterol:** 56 mg
	Sodium: 96 mg
Each serving with	**Fiber:** 3 g
potatoes provides:	**Protein:** 24 g
Calories: 274	**Carbohydrate:** 33 g
Total fat: 5 g	**Potassium:** 878 mg

Beef Casserole

Drain fat from cooked beef to lower the amount of fat and calories.

1/2 lb lean ground beef
1 cup onion, chopped
1 cup celery, chopped
1 cup green pepper, cubed
3 1/2 cups tomatoes, diced
1/4 tsp salt
1/2 tsp black pepper
1/4 tsp paprika
1 cup frozen peas
2 small carrots, diced
1 cup brown rice, uncooked
1 1/2 cups water

1. In a skillet, brown the ground beef and drain off the fat.
2. Add the rest of the ingredients. Mix well. Cook over medium heat and cover skillet until boiling. Reduce to low heat and simmer for 35 minutes. Serve hot.

Yield: 8 servings
Serving size: 1 1/3 cups

Each serving provides:
Calories: 201
Total fat: 5 g
Saturated fat: 2 g
Cholesterol: 16 mg

Sodium: 164 mg
Calcium: 33 mg
Iron: 2 mg
Fiber: 3 g
Protein: 9 g
Carbohydrate: 31 g
Potassium: 449 mg

Black Skillet Beef with Greens and Red Potatoes

This heart-healthy one-dish meal is made with lean top round beef, lots of vegetables, and a spicy, herb mixture.

1 lb top round beef
1 Tbsp paprika
1^1/$_2$ tsp oregano
^{1}/$_2$ tsp chili powder
^{1}/$_4$ tsp garlic powder
^{1}/$_4$ tsp black pepper
^{1}/$_8$ tsp red pepper
^{1}/$_8$ tsp dry mustard
8 red-skinned potatoes, halved
3 cups onion, finely chopped
2 cups beef broth
2 large garlic cloves, minced
2 large carrots, peeled and cut into very thin 2^1/$_2$-inch strips
2 bunches mustard greens, kale, or turnip greens, stems removed (^{1}/$_2$ lb each) and coarsely torn
non-stick spray coating as needed

1. Partially freeze beef. Thinly slice across the grain into long strips ^{1}/$_8$-inch thick and 3 inches wide. Trim away visible fat.
2. Combine paprika, oregano, chili powder, garlic powder, black pepper, red pepper, and dry mustard. Coat strips of meat with the spice mixture.
3. Spray a large heavy skillet with non-stick spray coating. Preheat pan over high heat.
4. Add meat; cook, stirring for 5 minutes.
5. Add potatoes, onion, broth, and garlic. Cook, covered, over medium heat, for 20 minutes.
6. Stir in carrots, lay greens over top, and cook, covered, until carrots are tender, about 15 minutes.
7. Serve in large serving bowl, with crusty bread for dunking.

Yield: 6 servings
Serving size: 7 oz

Each serving provides:
Calories: 340
Total fat: 5 g
Saturated fat: 2 g
Cholesterol: 64 mg
Sodium: 109 mg
Fiber: 8 g
Protein: 30 g
Carbohydrate: 45 g
Potassium: 1,278 mg

Shish Kabob

2 Tbsp olive oil
$1/2$ cup chicken broth
$1/4$ cup red wine
1 lemon, juice only
1 tsp garlic, chopped
$1/4$ tsp salt
$1/2$ tsp rosemary
$1/8$ tsp black pepper
2 lb lean lamb, cut into 1-inch cubes
24 cherry tomatoes
24 mushrooms
24 small onions

1. Combine oil, broth, wine, lemon juice, garlic, salt, rosemary, and pepper. Pour over lamb, tomatoes, mushrooms, and onions. Marinate in refrigerator for several hours or overnight.
2. Put together skewers of lamb, onions, mushrooms, and tomatoes. Broil 3 inches from heat for 15 minutes, turning every 5 minutes.

Yield: 8 servings
Serving size: 1 kabob, with 3 oz of meat

Each serving provides:
Calories: 274
Total fat: 12 g

Saturated fat: 3 g
Cholesterol: 75 mg
Sodium: 207 mg
Fiber: 3 g
Protein: 26 g
Carbohydrate: 16 g
Potassium: 728 mg

20-Minute Chicken Creole

This quick Southern dish contains no added fat and very little added salt in its spicy tomato sauce.

non-stick cooking spray as needed
4 medium chicken breast halves, skinned, boned, and cut into 1-inch strips*
1 can (14 oz) tomatoes, cut up**
1 cup chili sauce, low-sodium
1¹/₂ cups green peppers, chopped (1 large)
1¹/₂ cups celery, chopped
¹/₄ cup onion, chopped
2 cloves garlic, minced
1 Tbsp fresh basil or 1 tsp dried
1 Tbsp fresh parsley or 1 tsp dried
¹/₄ tsp crushed red pepper
¹/₄ tsp salt

1. Spray a deep skillet with non-stick spray coating. Preheat pan over high heat.
2. Cook chicken in hot skillet, stirring, for 3-5 minutes, or until no longer pink. Reduce heat.
3. Add tomatoes and their juice, low-sodium chili sauce, green pepper, celery, onion, garlic, basil, parsley, crushed red pepper, and salt. Bring to boiling; reduce heat and simmer, covered, for 10 minutes.
4. Serve over hot cooked rice or whole wheat pasta.

*For convenience, you can use uncooked boneless, skinless chicken breasts.

**To cut back on sodium, try low-sodium canned tomatoes.

Yield: 4 servings	**Cholesterol:** 73 mg
Serving size: 1¹/₂ cups	**Sodium:** 383 mg
	Fiber: 4 g
Each serving provides:	**Protein:** 30 g
Calories: 274	**Carbohydrate:** 30 g
Total fat: 5 g	**Potassium:** 944 mg
Saturated fat: 1 g	

Baked Chicken Nuggets

1¹/₂ lb chicken thighs, boneless and skinless
1 cup ready-to-eat cereal, cornflakes, crumbs
1 tsp paprika
¹/₂ tsp Italian herb seasoning
¹/₄ tsp garlic powder
¹/₄ tsp onion powder

1. Remove skin and bone; cut thighs into bite-size pieces.
2. Place cornflakes into plastic bag and crush by using a rolling pin.
3. Add remaining ingredients to crushed cornflakes. Close bag tightly and shake until blended.
4. Add a few chicken pieces at a time to crumb mixture. Shake to coat evenly.

Conventional Method
1. Preheat oven to 400° F. Lightly grease a cooking sheet.
2. Place chicken pieces on cooking sheet so they are not touching.
3. Bake until golden brown, about 12-14 minutes.

Note: To remove bone from chicken thighs:
1. Place chicken on cutting board. Remove skin from thighs.
2. Turn the chicken thighs over.
3. Cut around bone and remove it.

Yield: 4 servings
Serving size: about 3 oz

Each serving provides:
Calories: 175
Total fat: 8 g

Saturated fat: 2 g
Cholesterol: 67 mg
Sodium: 127 mg

≤ 30 mins   Entrées

Chicken Marsala

Wine, lemons, and mushrooms flavor this chicken recipe the lower-salt and lower-fat way.

¹/₈ tsp black pepper
¹/₄ tsp salt
¹/₄ cup flour
4 chicken breasts, boned, and skinless (5 oz)
1 Tbsp olive oil
¹/₂ cup Marsala wine
¹/₂ cup chicken stock, skim fat from top
¹/₂ lemon, fresh lemon juice
¹/₂ cup mushrooms, sliced
1 Tbsp fresh parsley, chopped

1. Mix together pepper, salt, and flour. Coat chicken with seasoned flour.
2. In a heavy-bottomed skillet, heat oil. Place chicken breasts in skillet and brown on both sides. Then remove chicken from skillet and set aside.
3. To the skillet, add wine and stir until the wine is heated. Add juice, stock, and mushrooms. Stir to toss, reduce heat, and cook for about 10 minutes until the sauce is partially reduced.
4. Return browned chicken breasts to skillet. Spoon sauce over the chicken.
5. Cover and cook for about 5-10 minutes or until chicken is done.
6. Serve sauce over chicken. Garnish with chopped parsley.

Yield: 4 servings
Serving size: 1 chicken breast with ¹/₃ cup sauce

Each serving provides:
Calories: 285
Total fat: 8 g
Saturated fat: 2 g
Cholesterol: 85 mg
Sodium: 236 mg
Fiber: 1 g
Protein: 33 g
Carbohydrate: 11 g
Potassium: 348 mg

≤ 30 mins   Entrées

Chicken Oriental

With no added salt and very little oil in the marinade, these broiled or grilled kabobs made with skinless chicken breasts are lower in saturated fat, cholesterol, and sodium.

8 chicken breasts, boneless and skinless
8 fresh mushrooms
black pepper to taste
8 whole white onions, parboiled
2 oranges, quartered
8 canned pineapple chunks
8 cherry tomatoes
1 can (6 oz) frozen, concentrated apple juice, thawed
1 cup dry white wine
2 Tbsp soy sauce, low-sodium
dash ground ginger
2 Tbsp vinegar
1/4 cup vegetable oil

1. Sprinkle chicken breasts with pepper.
2. Thread eight skewers as follows: chicken, mushroom, chicken, onion, chicken, orange quarter, chicken, pineapple chunk, cherry tomato.
3. Place kabobs into shallow pan.
4. Combine remaining ingredients; spoon over kabobs. Marinate in refrigerator at least 1 hour.
5. Drain. Broil 6 inches from heat, 15 minutes on each side, brushing with marinade every 5 minutes. Discard any leftover marinade.

Yield: 8 servings
Serving size: 1/2 chicken breast kabob

Each serving provides:
Calories: 359
Total fat: 11 g

Saturated fat: 2 g
Cholesterol: 66 mg
Sodium: 226 mg
Fiber: 3 g
Protein: 28 g
Carbohydrate: 34 g
Potassium: 756 mg

Chicken and Vegetables

1¹/₂ Tbsp margarine
1 tsp garlic powder
¹/₂ cup onions, chopped
1 lb 4 oz chicken thighs, boneless and skinless
10-oz package cut green beans, frozen
¹/₄ tsp pepper

1. Melt margarine in heavy skillet. Add garlic and onions; stir until blended. Cook over medium heat, until tender, about 5 minutes. Remove from skillet.
2. Place chicken in skillet. Cook over medium heat, until chicken is thoroughly done and no longer pink in color, about 12 minutes. Remove chicken from skillet; keep warm.
3. Place frozen green beans, pepper, and cooked onions in same skillet. Cover and cook over medium-low heat until beans are tender, about 5 minutes.
4. Add chicken to vegetable mixture. Continue cooking, stirring occasionally, until heated through, about 3 minutes.

Note: To remove bone from chicken thighs:
1. Place chicken on cutting board. Remove skin from thighs.
2. Turn the chicken thighs over.
3. Cut around bone and remove it.

Yield: 4 servings
Serving size: 1 cup

Each serving provides:
Calories: 190
Total fat: 11 g

Saturated fat: 3 g
Cholesterol: 57 mg
Sodium: 109 mg

Barbecued Chicken

3 lb chicken parts (breast, drumstick, and thigh), skin and fat removed
1 large onion
3 Tbsp vinegar
3 Tbsp Worcestershire sauce
2 Tbsp brown sugar
black pepper to taste
1 Tbsp hot pepper flakes
1 Tbsp chili powder
1 cup chicken stock or broth, fat skimmed from top

1. Place chicken into 13- by 9- by 2-inch pan. Arrange onions over top.
2. Mix together vinegar, Worcestershire sauce, brown sugar, pepper, hot pepper flakes, chili powder, and stock.
3. Pour mixture over chicken and bake at 350° F for 1 hour or until done. While cooking the chicken, baste occasionally.

Yield: 8 servings	**Saturated fat:** 2 g
Serving size: 1 chicken part with sauce	**Cholesterol:** 68 mg
	Sodium: 240 mg
	Fiber: 1 g
Each serving provides:	**Protein:** 24 g
Calories: 176	**Carbohydrate:** 7 g
Total fat: 6 g	**Potassium:** 360 mg

Chicken Ratatouille

Served over rice, this delicious dish is loaded with vegetables and skinless chicken breasts, making it a lower-fat, lower-salt one-dish meal.

1 Tbsp vegetable oil
4 medium chicken breast halves, skinned, fat removed, boned, and cut into 1-inch pieces
2 zucchini, about 7 inches long, unpeeled and thinly sliced
1 small eggplant, peeled and cut into 1-inch cubes
1 medium onion, thinly sliced
1 medium green pepper, cut into 1-inch pieces
1/2 lb fresh mushrooms, sliced
1 can (16 oz) whole tomatoes, cut up
1 clove garlic, minced
1 1/2 tsp dried basil, crushed
1 Tbsp fresh parsley, minced
black pepper to taste

1. Heat oil in large non-stick skillet. Add chicken and sauté about 3 minutes, or until lightly browned.
2. Add zucchini, eggplant, onion, green pepper, and mushrooms. Cook about 15 minutes, stirring occasionally.
3. Add tomatoes, garlic, basil, parsley, and pepper; stir and continue cooking about 5 minutes, or until chicken is tender.

Yield: 4 servings
Serving size: 1 1/2 cups

Each serving provides:
Calories: 266
Total fat: 8 g
Saturated fat: 2 g

Cholesterol: 66 mg
Sodium: 253 mg
Fiber: 6 g
Protein: 30 g
Carbohydrate: 21 g
Potassium: 1,148 mg

Chicken and Spanish Rice

1 cup onions, chopped
1/4 cup green peppers
2 tsp vegetable oil
1 can (8 oz) tomato sauce*
1 tsp parsley, chopped
1/2 tsp black pepper
11/4 tsp garlic, minced
5 cups brown rice, cooked in unsalted water
31/2 cups chicken breasts, cooked, skin and bone removed, and diced

1. In large skillet, sauté onions and green peppers in oil for 5 minutes on medium heat.
2. Add tomato sauce and spices. Heat through.
3. Add cooked rice and chicken. Heat through.

*Reduce sodium by using one 4-oz can of no-salt-added tomato sauce and one 4-oz can of regular tomato sauce. New sodium content for each serving is 226 mg.

Yield: 5 servings
Serving size: 11/2 cups

Each serving provides:
Calories: 428
Total fat: 52 g
Saturated fat: 2 g

Cholesterol: 80 mg
Sodium: 341 mg
Fiber: 8 g
Protein: 29 g
Carbohydrate: 35 g
Potassium: 545 mg

Chicken Stew

Save leftovers for lunch the next day.

8 chicken pieces (breasts or legs)
1 cup water
2 small garlic cloves, minced
1 small onion, chopped
1 1/2 tsp salt
1/2 tsp pepper
3 medium tomatoes, chopped
1 tsp parsley, chopped
1/4 cup celery, finely chopped
2 medium potatoes, peeled and chopped
2 small carrots, chopped
2 bay leaves

1. Remove the skin from the chicken and any extra fat. In a large skillet, combine chicken, water, garlic, onion, salt, pepper, tomatoes, and parsley. Tightly cover and cook over low heat for 25 minutes.
2. Add celery, potatoes, carrots, and bay leaves and continue to cook for 15 more minutes or until chicken and vegetables are tender. Remove bay leaves before serving.

Yield: 8 servings
Serving size: 1 piece of chicken

Each serving provides:
Calories: 206
Total fat: 6 g
Saturated fat: 2 g

Cholesterol: 75 mg
Sodium: 489 mg
Calcium: 32 mg
Iron: 2 mg
Protein: 28 g
Carbohydrate: 10 g
Potassium: 493 mg

Grilled Chicken with Green Chile Sauce

Marinate meats to make them tender without adding a lot of fat.

4 chicken breasts, skinless and boneless
1/4 cup olive oil
1/4 tsp oregano
1/2 tsp black pepper
1/4 cup water
10 to 12 tomatillos, husks removed and cut in half
1/2 medium onion, quartered
2 cloves garlic, finely chopped
2 serrano or jalapeno peppers
2 Tbsp cilantro, chopped
1/4 tsp salt
1/4 cup sour cream, low-fat
juice of 2 limes

1. Combine the oil, juice from one lime, oregano, and black pepper in a shallow glass baking dish. Stir. Place the chicken breasts in the baking dish and turn to coat each side. Cover the dish and refrigerate overnight. Turn the chicken periodically to marinate chicken on both sides.

2. Put water, tomatillos, and onion into a saucepan. Bring to a gentle boil and cook, uncovered, for 10 minutes or until the tomatillos are tender. In a blender, place the cooked onion, tomatillos, and any remaining water. Add the garlic, peppers, cilantro, salt, and the remaining lime juice. Blend until all ingredients are smooth. Place the sauce into a bowl and refrigerate.

3. Place the chicken breasts on a hot grill and cook until done. Place the chicken on a serving platter.

4. Spoon a tablespoon of low-fat sour cream over each chicken breast. Pour the sauce over the sour cream.

Yield: 4 servings	**Cholesterol:** 73 mg
Serving size: 1 breast	**Sodium:** 91 mg
	Calcium: 53 mg
Each serving	**Iron:** 2 mg
provides:	**Fiber:** 3 g
Calories: 210	**Protein:** 29 g
Total fat: 5 g	**Carbohydrate:** 14 g
Saturated fat: 1 g	**Potassium:** 780 mg

Chicken and Rice

Take the skin off chicken to lower saturated fat and calories.

6 chicken pieces (legs and breasts), skinned
2 tsp vegetable oil
4 cups water
2 tomatoes, chopped
$1/2$ cup green pepper, chopped
$1/4$ cup red pepper, chopped
$1/4$ cup celery, diced
1 medium carrot, grated
$1/4$ cup corn, frozen
$1/2$ cup onion, chopped
$1/4$ cup fresh cilantro, chopped
2 cloves garlic, finely chopped
$1/8$ tsp salt
$1/8$ tsp pepper
2 cups brown rice
$1/2$ cup peas, frozen
2 oz Spanish olives
$1/4$ cup raisins

1. In a large pot, brown chicken pieces in oil.
2. Add water, tomatoes, green and red peppers, celery, carrots, corn, onion, cilantro, garlic, salt, and pepper. Cover and cook over medium heat for 20-30 minutes or until chicken is done.
3. Remove chicken from the pot and place in the refrigerator. Add rice, peas, and olives to the pot. Cover pot and cook over low heat for about 20 minutes until rice is cooked.
4. Add chicken and raisins and cook for another 8 minutes.

(continued)

Chicken and Rice (continued)

Yield: 6 servings
Serving size: 1 cup of rice and 1 piece of chicken

Each serving provides:
Calories: 448
Total fat: 7 g
Saturated fat: 2 g

Cholesterol: 49 mg
Sodium: 352 mg
Calcium: 63 mg
Iron: 4 mg
Fiber: 4 g
Protein: 24 g
Carbohydrate: 70 g
Potassium: 551 mg

Spicy Southern Barbecued Chicken

Removing the chicken fat and skin and adding no salt to the tasty sauce makes this chicken favorite heart-healthy.

5 Tbsp (3 oz) tomato paste
1 tsp ketchup
2 tsp honey
1 tsp molasses
1 tsp Worcestershire sauce
4 tsp white vinegar
$3/4$ tsp cayenne pepper
$1/8$ tsp black pepper
$1/4$ tsp onion powder
2 cloves garlic, minced
$1/8$ tsp ginger, grated
$1^1/2$ lb chicken (breasts and drumsticks), skinless

1. Combine all ingredients except chicken in saucepan.
2. Simmer for 15 minutes.
3. Place chicken on large platter and brush with half of sauce mixture.
4. Cover with plastic wrap and marinate in refrigerator for 1 hour.
5. Place chicken on baking sheet lined with aluminum foil and broil for 10 minutes on each side to seal in juices.
6. Turn oven to 350° F and add remaining sauce to chicken. Cover chicken with aluminum foil and continue baking for 30 minutes.

Yield: 6 servings
Serving size: $1/2$ breast or 2 small drumsticks

Each serving provides:
Calories: 176
Total fat: 4 g
Saturated fat: less than 1 g

Cholesterol: 81 mg
Sodium: 199 mg
Fiber: 1 g
Protein: 27 g
Carbohydrate: 7 g
Potassium: 392 mg

≤ 90 mins   Entrées

Yosemite Chicken Stew and Dumplings

Skinless chicken is the basis of this delicious stew with cornmeal dumplings made with low-fat milk.

For the stew:

1 lb chicken meat, skinless, boneless, and cut into 1-inch cubes
1/2 cup onion, coarsely chopped
1 medium carrot, peeled and thinly sliced
1 stalk celery, thinly sliced
1/4 tsp salt
black pepper to taste
1 pinch ground cloves
1 bay leaf
3 cups water
1 tsp cornstarch
1 tsp dried basil
1 package (10 oz) frozen peas

For the cornmeal dumplings:

1 cup yellow cornmeal
3/4 cup all-purpose flour, sifted
2 tsp baking powder
1/2 tsp salt
1 cup milk, low-fat (1%)
1 Tbsp vegetable oil

For the stew:

1. Place chicken, onion, carrot, celery, salt, pepper, cloves, bay leaf, and water into a large saucepan. Heat to boiling; cover and reduce heat to simmer. Cook about 1/2 hour or until chicken is tender.
2. Remove chicken and vegetables from broth. Strain broth.

(continued)

Yosemite Chicken Stew and Dumplings (continued)

3. Skim fat from broth; measure and, if necessary, add water to make 3 cups of liquid.
4. Mix cornstarch with 1 cup cooled broth by shaking vigorously in a jar with a tight-fitting lid.
5. Pour into saucepan with remaining broth; cook, stirring constantly, until mixture comes to a boil and is thickened.
6. Add basil, peas, and reserved vegetables to sauce; stir to combine.
7. Add chicken and heat slowly to boiling while preparing cornmeal dumplings.

For the dumplings:
1. Sift together cornmeal, flour, baking powder, and salt into a large mixing bowl.
2. Mix together milk and oil. Add milk mixture all at once to dry ingredients; stir just enough to moisten flour and to evenly distribute liquid. Dough will be soft.
3. Drop by full tablespoons on top of braised meat or stew. Cover tightly; heat to boiling. Reduce heat (do not lift cover) to simmering and steam about 20 minutes.

Yield: 6 servings
Serving size: 1¼ cups stew with 2 dumplings

Each serving provides:
Calories: 301
Total fat: 6 g

Saturated fat: 1 g
Cholesterol: 43 mg
Sodium: 471 mg
Fiber: 5 g
Protein: 24 g
Carbohydrate: 37 g
Potassium: 409 mg

Turkey Patties

1 lb 4 oz ground turkey
1 cup bread crumbs
1 egg
1/4 cup green onions, chopped
1 Tbsp prepared mustard
1 1/2 Tbsp margarine
1/2 cup chicken broth

1. Mix ground turkey, bread crumbs, egg, onions, and mustard in large bowl. Shape into four patties, about 1/2-inch thick.
2. Melt margarine in large skillet over low heat. Add patties and cook, turning once to brown other side. Cook until golden brown outside and white inside, about 10 minutes. Remove from skillet and place on plate.
3. Add chicken broth to skillet, and boil over high heat until slightly thickened, about 1-2 minutes. Pour sauce over patties.
4. Serve on buns.

Yield: 4 servings
Serving size: 1 patty

Each serving provides:
Calories: 305
Total fat: 18 g

Saturated fat: 5 g
Cholesterol: 149 mg
Sodium: 636 mg

≤ 30 mins   Entrées

Turkey Stir-Fry

1 chicken bouillon cube
$^1/_2$ cup hot water
2 Tbsp soy sauce
1 Tbsp cornstarch
2 Tbsp vegetable oil
$^1/_2$ tsp garlic powder
1 lb turkey, cubed
$1^3/_4$ cups carrots, thinly sliced
1 cup zucchini, sliced
$^1/_2$ cup onions, thinly sliced
$^1/_4$ cup hot water

1. Combine chicken bouillon cube and hot water to make broth; stir until dissolved.
2. Combine broth, soy sauce, and cornstarch in small bowl. Set aside.
3. Heat oil in skillet over high heat. Add garlic and turkey. Cook, stirring, until turkey is thoroughly cooked and no longer pink in color.
4. Add carrots, zucchini, onion, and water to cooked turkey. Cover and cook, stirring occasionally, until vegetables are tender-crisp, about 5 minutes. Uncover; bring turkey mixture to boil. Cook until almost all liquid has evaporated.
5. Stir in cornstarch mixture. Bring to boil, stirring constantly until thickened.

Note: Serve over steamed rice.

Yield: 4 servings
Serving size: $^1/_2$ cup

Each serving provides:
Calories: 195
Total fat: 9 g

Saturated fat: 2 g
Cholesterol: 44 mg
Sodium: 506 mg

Spaghetti with Turkey Meat Sauce

Using non-stick cooking spray, ground turkey, and no added salt helps to make this classic dish heart-healthy.

non-stick cooking spray as needed
1 lb ground turkey
1 can (28 oz) tomatoes, cut up
1 cup green pepper, finely chopped
1 cup onion, finely chopped
2 cloves garlic, minced
1 tsp dried oregano, crushed
1 tsp black pepper
1 lb spaghetti, uncooked

1. Spray a large skillet with non-stick spray coating. Preheat over high heat.
2. Add turkey; cook, stirring occasionally, for 5 minutes. Drain fat and discard.
3. Stir in tomatoes with their juice, green pepper, onion, garlic, oregano, and black pepper. Bring to a boil; reduce heat. Simmer covered for 15 minutes, stirring occasionally. Remove cover; simmer for 15 minutes more. (If you like a creamier sauce, give sauce a whirl in your blender or food processor.)
4. Meanwhile, cook spaghetti in unsalted water. Drain well.
5. Serve sauce over spaghetti.

Yield: 6 servings
Serving size: 5 oz sauce and 9 oz spaghetti

Each serving provides:
Calories: 455
Total fat: 6 g

Saturated fat: 1 g
Cholesterol: 51 mg
Sodium: 248 mg
Fiber: 5 g
Protein: 28 g
Carbohydrate: 71 g
Potassium: 593 mg

≤ 60 mins   Entrées

Turkey Meatloaf

Here's a healthier version of an old diner favorite.

1 lb lean ground turkey
$^1/_2$ cup regular oats, dry
1 large egg
1 Tbsp onion, dehydrated
$^1/_4$ cup ketchup

1. Combine all ingredients and mix well.
2. Bake in loaf pan at 350° F or to internal temperature of 165° F for 25 minutes.
3. Cut into 5 slices and serve.

Yield: 5 servings   Cholesterol: 102 mg
Serving size: 1 slice   Sodium: 205 mg
                                   Fiber: 1 g
Each serving provides: Protein: 22 g
Calories: 191   Carbohydrate: 9 g
Total fat: 7 g   Potassium: 268 mg
Saturated fat: 2 g

Turkey Stuffed Cabbage

This hearty entrée uses half ground turkey and half lean ground beef and no added salt for a lower in fat and salt taste treat.

1 head cabbage
1/2 lb lean ground beef
1/2 lb ground turkey
1 small onion, minced
1 slice stale whole wheat bread, crumbled
1/4 cup water
1/8 tsp black pepper
1 can (16 oz) diced tomatoes
1 small onion, sliced
1 cup water
1 medium carrot, sliced
1 Tbsp lemon juice
2 Tbsp brown sugar
1 Tbsp cornstarch

1. Rinse and core cabbage. Carefully remove 10 outer leaves, place in saucepan, and cover with boiling water. Simmer 5 minutes. Remove and drain cooked cabbage leaves on paper towels.
2. Shred 1/2 cup of raw cabbage and set aside.
3. Brown ground beef and turkey and minced onion in skillet. Drain fat.
4. Place cooked and drained meat mixture, bread crumbs, water, and pepper into mixing bowl.
5. Drain tomatoes, reserving liquid, and add 1/2 cup of tomato juice from can to meat mixture. Mix well; then place 1/4 cup of filling on each parboiled, drained cabbage leaf. Place folded side down in skillet.

(continued)

Turkey Stuffed Cabbage (continued)

6. Add tomatoes, sliced onion, water, shredded cabbage, and carrot. Cover and simmer about 1 hour (or until cabbage is tender), basting occasionally.
7. Remove cabbage rolls to serving platter; keep warm.
8. Mix lemon juice, brown sugar, and cornstarch together in small bowl. Add to vegetables and liquid in skillet, and cook, stirring occasionally, until thickened and clear. Serve over cabbage rolls.

Yield: 5 servings	**Cholesterol:** 56 mg
Serving size: 2 rolls each	**Sodium:** 235 mg
	Fiber: 3 g
Each serving provides:	**Protein:** 20 g
Calories: 235	**Carbohydrate:** 18 g
Total fat: 9 g	**Potassium:** 545 mg
Saturated fat: 3 g	

Baked Salmon Dijon

1 cup sour cream, fat-free
2 tsp dried dill
3 Tbsp scallions, finely chopped
2 Tbsp Dijon mustard
2 Tbsp lemon juice
1 1/2 lb salmon fillet with skin, cut in center
1/2 tsp garlic powder
1/2 tsp black pepper
fat-free cooking spray as needed

1. Whisk sour cream, dill, onion, mustard, and lemon juice in small bowl to blend.
2. Preheat oven to 400° F. Lightly oil baking sheet with cooking spray.
3. Place salmon, skin side down, on prepared sheet. Sprinkle with garlic powder and pepper, then spread with the sauce.
4. Bake salmon until just opaque in center, about 20 minutes.

Yield: 6 servings
Serving size: 1 piece
(4 oz)

Each serving provides:
Calories: 196
Total fat: 7 g

Saturated fat: 2 g
Cholesterol: 76 mg
Sodium: 229 mg
Fiber: less than 1 g
Protein: 27 g
Carbohydrate: 5 g
Potassium: 703 mg

Baked Trout Olé
Bake fish with only a small amount of oil.

2 lb trout fillet, cut into 6 pieces (any kind of fish can be used)
3 Tbsp lime juice (about 2 limes)
1 medium tomato, chopped
1/2 medium onion, chopped
3 Tbsp cilantro, chopped
1/2 tsp olive oil
1/4 tsp black pepper
1/4 tsp salt
1/4 tsp red pepper (optional)

1. Preheat oven to 350° F.
2. Rinse fish and pat dry. Place into baking dish.
3. In a separate dish, mix remaining ingredients together and pour over fish.
4. Bake for 15-20 minutes or until fork-tender.

Yield: 6 servings
Serving size: 1 piece

Each serving provides:
Calories: 236
Fat: 9 g
Saturated fat: 3 g
Cholesterol: 104 mg

Sodium: 197 mg
Calcium: 60 mg
Iron: 1 mg
Fiber: less than 1 g
Protein: 34 g
Carbohydrate: 2 g
Potassium: 865 mg

Scallop Kabobs

These colorful skewers contain scallops, which are naturally low in total and saturated fat.

3 medium green peppers, cut into 1¹/₂-inch squares
1¹/₂ lb fresh bay scallops
1 pt cherry tomatoes
¹/₄ cup dry white wine
¹/₄ cup vegetable oil
3 Tbsp lemon juice
dash garlic powder
black pepper to taste

1. Parboil green peppers for 2 minutes.
2. Alternately thread first three ingredients on skewers.
3. Combine next five ingredients.
4. Brush kabobs with wine, oil, and lemon mixture; place on grill (or under broiler).
5. Grill 15 minutes, turning and basting frequently.

Yield: 4 servings
Serving size: 6-oz scallop kabob

Each serving provides:
Calories: 224
Fat: 6 g

Saturated fat: 1 g
Cholesterol: 43 mg
Sodium: 355 mg
Fiber: 3 g
Protein: 30 g
Carbohydrate: 13 g
Potassium: 993 mg

Spicy Baked Fish

1 lb salmon (or other fish) fillet
1 Tbsp olive oil
1 tsp spicy seasoning, salt-free

1. Preheat oven to 350° F. Spray a casserole dish with cooking oil spray.
2. Wash and dry fish. Place in dish. Mix oil and seasoning, and drizzle over fish.
3. Bake uncovered for 15 minutes or until fish flakes with fork. Cut into four pieces. Serve with rice.

Yield: 4 servings
Serving size: 1 piece
(3 oz)

Each serving provides:
Calories: 192
Fat: 11 g

Saturated fat: 2 g
Cholesterol: 63 mg
Sodium: 50 mg
Fiber: 0 g
Protein: 23 g
Carbohydrate: 23 g
Potassium: 560 mg

Catfish Stew and Rice

2 medium potatoes
1 can (14¹/₂ oz) tomatoes, cut up*
1 cup onion, chopped
1 cup (8-oz bottle) clam juice or water
1 cup water
2 cloves garlic, minced
¹/₂ head cabbage, coarsely chopped
1 lb catfish fillets
green onion, sliced, as needed
1¹/₂ Tbsp Chili and Spice Seasoning (see recipe on page 126)
2 cups rice (brown or white), cooked

Reduce the sodium by using low- or no-added-sodium canned tomatoes.

1. Peel potatoes and cut into quarters.
2. In large pot, combine potatoes, tomatoes and their juice, onion, clam juice, water, and garlic. Bring to boil and reduce heat. Cook covered over medium-low heat for 10 minutes.
3. Add cabbage and return to boil. Reduce heat. Cook covered over medium-low heat for 5 minutes, stirring occasionally.
4. Meanwhile, cut fillets into 2-inch lengths. Coat with Chili and Spice Seasoning.
5. Add fish to vegetables. Reduce heat and simmer covered for 5 minutes or until fish flakes easily with fork.
6. Serve in soup plates. Garnish with sliced green onion, if desired. Serve with scoop of hot cooked rice.

Yield: 4 servings	**Saturated fat:** 2 g
Serving size: 1 cup of stew with ¹/₂ cup of rice	**Cholesterol:** 87 mg
	Sodium: 355 mg
	Fiber: 4 g
Each serving provides:	**Protein:** 28 g
Calories: 363	**Carbohydrate:** 44 g
Total fat: 8 g	**Potassium:** 1,079 mg

Mediterranean Baked Fish

This dish is baked and flavored with a Mediterranean-style tomato, onion, and garlic sauce to make it lower in fat and salt.

2 tsp olive oil
1 large onion, sliced
1 can (16 oz) whole tomatoes, drained (reserve juice) and coarsely chopped
1 bay leaf
1 clove garlic, minced
1 cup dry white wine
1/2 cup reserved tomato juice, from canned tomatoes
1/4 cup lemon juice
1/4 cup orange juice
1 Tbsp fresh orange peel, grated
1 tsp fennel seeds, crushed
1/2 tsp dried oregano, crushed
1/2 tsp dried thyme, crushed
1/2 tsp dried basil, crushed
black pepper to taste
1 lb fish fillets (sole, flounder, salmon, or sea perch)

1. Heat oil in large non-stick skillet. Add onion, and sauté over moderate heat 5 minutes or until soft.
2. Add all remaining ingredients except fish.
3. Stir well and simmer 30 minutes, uncovered.
4. Arrange fish in a 10- by 6-inch baking dish; cover with sauce.
5. Bake, uncovered, at 375° F about 15 minutes or until fish flakes easily.

Yield: 4 servings
Serving size: 4-oz fillet with sauce

Each serving provides:
Calories: 178
Total fat: 4 g
Saturated fat: 1 g
Cholesterol: 56 mg
Sodium: 260 mg
Fiber: 3 g
Protein: 22 g
Carbohydrate: 12 g
Potassium: 678 mg

Mouth-Watering Oven-Fried Fish

For variety, try this heart-healthy fish recipe with any kind of fish.

2 lb fish fillets
1 Tbsp fresh lemon juice
$^1/_4$ cup milk, fat-free or
buttermilk, low-fat
2 drops hot pepper sauce
1 tsp fresh garlic, minced
$^1/_4$ tsp white pepper, ground
$^1/_4$ tsp salt
$^1/_4$ tsp onion powder
$^1/_2$ cup cornflakes, crumbled, or regular bread crumbs
1 Tbsp vegetable oil (for greasing baking dish)
1 fresh lemon, cut into wedges

1. Preheat oven to 475° F.
2. Wipe fillets with lemon juice and pat dry.
3. Combine milk, hot pepper sauce, and garlic.
4. Combine pepper, salt, and onion powder with cornflake crumbs and place on a plate.
5. Let fillets sit in milk briefly. Remove and coat fillets on both sides with seasoned crumbs. Let stand briefly until coating sticks to each side of fish.
6. Arrange on lightly oiled shallow baking dish.
7. Bake 20 minutes on middle rack without turning.
8. Cut into six pieces. Serve with fresh lemon.

Yield: 6 servings
Serving size: 1 cut piece

Each serving provides:
Calories: 183
Total fat: 2 g
Saturated fat: 1 g

Cholesterol: 80 mg
Sodium: 325 mg
Fiber: 1 g
Protein: 30 g
Carbohydrate: 10 g
Potassium: 453 mg

Frittata Primavera

3 tsp olive oil
1/4 cup onion, chopped
1 clove garlic, finely chopped
1/2 cup fresh asparagus pieces
1/2 cup canned or frozen artichoke hearts, chopped
1/2 cup sugar snap peas, strings pulled and cut into 1/2-inch pieces
1/4 tsp dried basil
salt and pepper to taste
3/4 cup egg substitute or 3 eggs
1 Tbsp plain yogurt, low-fat
1 Tbsp Parmesan cheese, grated

1. Heat 1 teaspoon of the oil in a skillet and cook the onion 2 or 3 minutes or until soft.
2. Add the garlic and cook 1 minute more.
3. Stir in the asparagus, artichoke hearts, peas, basil, and pepper, and cook, stirring occasionally until tender but still slightly crisp, 3-5 minutes. Set aside.
4. Preheat the broiler.
5. Beat the egg substitute or eggs with the yogurt and another pinch of pepper.
6. Heat the remaining oil in a heavy-bottom skillet. Pour in the egg mixture and cook until just set on the bottom but still wet on the top, 1 minute.
7. Scatter the vegetables over the top and set into the oven to finish cooking, 2 minutes.
8. Dust the top with the Parmesan cheese, grated, and serve.

Yield: 2 servings

Each serving provides:
Calories: 126
Total fat: 3 g
Saturated fat: 1 g
Carbohydrate: 11 g
Sodium: 388 mg
Fiber: 2 g

Classic Macaroni and Cheese

Low-fat cheese and skim milk help to make this favorite dish heart-healthy.

2 cups macaroni
1/2 cup onions, chopped
1/2 cup evaporated milk, fat-free
1 medium egg, beaten
1/4 tsp black pepper
1 1/4 cups sharp cheddar cheese (4 oz), finely shredded, low-fat
non-stick cooking oil spray

1. Cook macaroni according to directions. (Do not add salt to the cooking water.) Drain and set aside.
2. Spray a casserole dish with non-stick cooking oil spray. Preheat oven to 350° F.
3. Lightly spray saucepan with non-stick cooking oil spray.
4. Add onions to saucepan and sauté for about 3 minutes.
5. In another bowl, combine macaroni, onions, and the remaining ingredients and mix thoroughly.
6. Transfer mixture into casserole dish.
7. Bake for 25 minutes or until bubbly. Let stand for 10 minutes before serving.

Yield: 8 servings
Serving size: 1/2 cup

Each serving provides:
Calories: 200
Total fat: 4 g
Saturated fat: 2 g

Cholesterol: 34 mg
Sodium: 120 mg
Fiber: 1 g
Protein: 11 g
Carbohydrate: 29 g
Potassium: 119 mg

Parmesan Rice and Pasta Pilaf

After the pasta and onion are sautéed, the oil is drained to minimize the fat content of this interesting pilaf.

2 Tbsp olive oil
1/2 cup vermicelli, uncooked and finely broken
2 Tbsp onion, diced
1 cup long-grain white or brown rice, uncooked
1 1/4 cups hot chicken stock
1 1/4 cups hot water
1/4 tsp ground white pepper
1 bay leaf
2 Tbsp Parmesan cheese, grated

1. In a large skillet, heat oil. Sauté vermicelli and onion until golden brown, about 2-4 minutes over medium-high heat. Drain off oil.
2. Add rice, stock, water, pepper, and bay leaf. Cover and simmer 15-20 minutes. Fluff with fork. Cover and let stand 5-20 minutes. Remove bay leaf.
3. Sprinkle with Parmesan cheese and serve immediately.

Yield: 6 servings	**Cholesterol:** 2 mg
Serving size: 2/3 cup	**Sodium:** 140 mg
	Fiber: 1 g
Each serving provides:	**Protein:** 5 g
Calories: 208	**Carbohydrate:** 33 g
Total fat: 6 g	**Potassium:** 90 mg
Saturated fat: 1 g	

Summer Vegetable Spaghetti

This lively vegetarian pasta dish contains no added fat or oil, is low in cholesterol, and is good hot or cold.

2 cups small yellow onions, cut into eighths
2 cups fresh ripe tomatoes (about 1 lb), chopped and peeled
2 cups yellow and green squash (about 1 lb), thinly sliced
1^1/$_2$ cups fresh green beans (about ^{1}/$_2$ lb), cut
^{2}/$_3$ cup water
2 Tbsp fresh parsley, minced
1 clove garlic, minced
^{1}/$_2$ tsp chili powder
^{1}/$_4$ tsp salt
black pepper to taste
1 can (6 oz) tomato paste
1 lb spaghetti, uncooked
^{1}/$_2$ cup Parmesan cheese, grated

1. Combine first 10 ingredients in large saucepan; cook for 10 minutes, then stir in tomato paste. Cover and cook gently, 15 minutes, stirring occasionally until vegetables are tender.
2. Cook spaghetti in unsalted water according to package directions.
3. Spoon sauce over drained hot spaghetti and sprinkle Parmesan cheese over top.

Yield: 9 servings
Serving size: 1 cup spaghetti and ^{3}/$_4$ cup sauce with vegetables

Each serving provides:
Calories: 271
Total fat: 3 g
Saturated fat: 1 g
Cholesterol: 4 mg
Sodium: 328 mg
Fiber: 5 g
Protein: 11 g
Carbohydrate: 51 g
Potassium: 436 mg

Vegetarian Spaghetti Sauce

2 Tbsp olive oil
2 small onions, chopped
3 cloves garlic, chopped
1¼ cups zucchini, sliced
1 Tbsp oregano, dried
1 Tbsp basil, dried
1 can (8-oz) tomato sauce
1 can (6-oz) tomato paste*
2 medium tomatoes, chopped
1 cup water

1. In a medium skillet, heat oil. Sauté onions, garlic, and zucchini in oil for 5 minutes on medium heat.
2. Add remaining ingredients and simmer covered for 45 minutes. Serve over spaghetti.

*To reduce sodium, use a 6-oz can of no-salt-added tomato paste. New sodium content for each serving is 260 mg.

Yield: 6 servings
Serving size: ³/₄ cup

Each serving provides:
Calories: 105
Total fat: 5 g
Saturated fat: 1 g
Cholesterol: 0 mg

Sodium: 479 mg
Fiber: 4 g
Protein: 3 g
Carbohydrate: 15 g
Potassium: 686 mg

≤ 90 mins   Entrées

Italian Vegetable Bake

This colorful low-sodium cholesterol-free vegetable baked dish is prepared without any added fat.

1 can (28 oz) whole tomatoes
1 medium onion, sliced
$^1/_2$ lb fresh green beans, sliced
$^1/_2$ lb fresh okra, cut into $^1/_2$-inch pieces, or $^3/_4$ cup or $^1/_2$ 10-oz package frozen okra
$^3/_4$ cup green pepper, finely chopped
2 Tbsp lemon juice
1 tsp fresh basil, chopped, or 1 tsp dried basil, crushed
$1^1/_2$ tsp fresh oregano leaves, chopped, or $^1/_2$ tsp dried oregano, crushed
3 medium (7-inch-long) zucchini, cut into 1-inch cubes
1 medium eggplant, pared and cut into 1-inch cubes
2 Tbsp Parmesan cheese, grated

1. Drain and coarsely chop tomatoes. Save liquid. Mix together tomatoes and reserved liquid, onion, green beans, okra, green pepper, lemon juice, and herbs. Cover and bake at 325° F for 15 minutes.
2. Mix in zucchini and eggplant, and continue baking, covered, 60-70 more minutes or until vegetables are tender. Stir occasionally.
3. Sprinkle top with Parmesan cheese just before serving.

Yield: 18 servings	**Sodium:** 86 mg
Serving size: $^1/_2$ cup	**Fiber:** 2 g
	Protein: 2 g
Each serving provides:	**Carbohydrate:** 5 g
Calories: 27	**Potassium:** 244 mg
Total fat: less than 1 g	
Saturated fat: less than 1 g	
Cholesterol: 1 mg	

Vegetable Stew

This stew is a great way to use summer vegetables in a new way.

3 cups water
1 cube vegetable bouillon, low-sodium
2 cups white potatoes, cut into 2-inch strips
2 cups carrots, sliced
4 cups summer squash, cut into 1-inch squares
1 cup summer squash, cut into 4 chunks
1 can (15 oz) sweet corn, rinsed and drained, or 2 ears fresh corn, 1¹/₂ cups
1 tsp thyme
2 cloves garlic, minced
1 stalk scallion, chopped
¹/₂ small hot pepper, chopped
1 cup onion, coarsely chopped
1 cup tomatoes, diced
(Add other favorite vegetables such as broccoli and cauliflower)

1. Heat water and bouillon in a large pot and bring to a boil.
2. Add potatoes and carrots to the broth and simmer for 5 minutes.
3. Add the remaining ingredients except for the tomatoes, and continue cooking for 15 minutes over medium heat.
4. Remove four chunks of squash and purée in blender.
5. Return puréed mixture to pot and let cook for 10 minutes more.
6. Add tomatoes and cook for another 5 minutes.
7. Remove from flame and let sit for minutes to allow stew to thicken.

Yield: 8 servings
Serving size: 1¹/₄ cups

Each serving provides:
Calories: 119
Total fat: 1 g
Saturated fat: less than 1 g

Cholesterol: 0 g
Sodium: 196 mg
Fiber: 4 g
Protein: 4 g
Carbohydrate: 27 g
Potassium: 524 mg

≤ 90 mins   Entrées

Zucchini Lasagna

Say, "Cheese," because this healthy version of a favorite comfort food will leave you smiling.

¹/₂ lb lasagna noodles, cooked in unsalted water
³/₄ cup part-skim mozzarella cheese, grated
1¹/₂ cups cottage cheese,* fat-free
¹/₄ cup Parmesan cheese, grated
1¹/₂ cups raw zucchini, sliced
2¹/₂ cups no-salt-added tomato sauce
2 tsp basil, dried
2 tsp oregano, dried
¹/₄ cup onion, chopped
1 clove garlic
¹/₈ tsp black pepper

1. Preheat oven to 350° F. Lightly spray 9- by 13-inch baking dish with vegetable oil spray.
2. In small bowl, combine ¹/₈ cup of mozzarella and 1 tablespoon of Parmesan cheese. Set aside.
3. In medium bowl, combine remaining mozzarella and Parmesan cheese with all the cottage cheese. Mix well and set aside.
4. Combine tomato sauce with remaining ingredients. Spread thin layer of tomato sauce in bottom of baking dish. Add a third of the noodles in a single layer. Spread half of cottage cheese mixture on top. Add layer of zucchini.
5. Repeat layering. Add thin coating of sauce. Top with noodles, sauce, and reserved cheese mixture. Cover with aluminum foil.
6. Bake for 30-40 minutes. Cool for 10-15 minutes. Cut into six portions.

Use unsalted cottage cheese to reduce the sodium content. New sodium content for each serving is 196 mg.

(continued)

Zucchini Lasagna (continued)

Yield: 6 servings
Serving size: 1 piece

Each serving provides:
Calories: 200
Total fat: 5 g
Saturated fat: 3 g

Cholesterol: 12 g
Sodium: 368 mg
Fiber: 3 g
Protein: 15 g
Carbohydrate: 24 g
Potassium: 593 mg

Brown or White Rice

Only 1 tablespoon of oil is used in this tasty and heart-healthy rice dish.

1 Tbsp vegetable oil
$^1/_2$ medium onion, chopped
2 cloves garlic, minced
2 cups long-grain brown or white rice
4 cups hot water
$^1/_2$ tsp salt
$^1/_2$ cup corn, peas, carrots, or peppers (optional), fresh or frozen

1. In medium pan, heat oil and sauté onion, garlic, and rice. Add hot water and salt. Bring to a full boil. Cover and simmer for 15 minutes without stirring. If desired, add vegetables, cover, and cook for an additional 5 minutes.
2. Uncover, give rice a full turn, and cover again. Turn heat off.
3. Let stand 15 minutes before serving.

Yield: 6 servings
Serving size: $^1/_2$ cup

Each serving provides:
Calories: 270
Total fat: 3 g

Saturated fat: less than 1 g
Cholesterol: 0 g
Sodium: 21 mg
Calcium: 28 mg
Iron: 2 mg

≤ 30 mins   Sides

Caribbean Pink Beans
Make beans without lard or other fat.

1 lb pink beans
10 cups water
2 medium plantains, finely chopped
1 large tomato, finely chopped
1 small red pepper, finely chopped
1 medium white onion, finely chopped
3 cloves garlic, finely chopped
1¹/₂ tsp salt

1. Rinse and pick through the beans. Put the beans into a large pot and add 10 cups of water. Place the pot into the refrigerator and allow the beans to soak overnight.
2. Cook the beans until they are soft. Add more water as needed while the beans are cooking.
3. Add the plantains, tomato, pepper, onion, garlic, and salt. Continue cooking at low heat until the plantains are soft.

Option: Serve with rice.

Yield: 16 servings	**Sodium:** 205 mg
Serving size: ¹/₂ cup	**Calcium:** 39 mg
	Iron: 2 mg
Each serving provides:	**Fiber:** 5 g
Calories: 133	**Protein:** 6 g
Total fat: less than 1 g	**Carbohydrate:** 28 g
Saturated fat: less than 1 g	**Potassium:** 495 mg
Cholesterol: 0 g	

≤ 30 mins   Sides

Green Beans Sauté

Green beans and onions are lightly sautéed in only 1 tablespoon of oil.

1 lb green beans, fresh or frozen, cut into 1-inch pieces
1 Tbsp vegetable oil
1 large yellow onion, halved lengthwise and thinly sliced
1/2 tsp salt
1/8 tsp black pepper
1 Tbsp fresh parsley, minced

1. If using fresh green beans, cook green beans in boiling water for 10-12 minutes or steam for 2-3 minutes until barely fork-tender. Drain well. If using frozen green beans, thaw first.
2. Heat oil in a large skillet. Sauté onion until golden.
3. Stir in green beans, salt, and pepper. Heat through.
4. Toss with parsley before serving.

Yield: 4 servings
Serving size: 3/4 cup

Each serving provides:
Calories: 64
Total fat: 4 g
Saturated fat: less than 1 g

Cholesterol: 0 g
Sodium: 282 mg
Fiber: 3 g
Protein: 2 g
Carbohydrate: 8 g
Potassium: 161 mg

Oriental Rice

Skimming the fat off the chicken stock and using a minimum of oil and no added salt means that this crunchy rice is lower in fat, saturated fat, and sodium.

1¹/₂ cups water
1 cup chicken stock or broth, skim fat from top
1¹/₃ cups long-grain white or brown rice, uncooked
2 tsp vegetable oil
2 Tbsp onion, finely chopped
2 Tbsp green pepper, finely chopped
¹/₂ cup pecans, chopped
¹/₄ tsp ground sage
1 cup celery, finely chopped
¹/₂ cup water chestnuts, sliced
¹/₄ tsp nutmeg
black pepper to taste

1. Bring water and stock to a boil in medium-size saucepan.
2. Add rice and stir. Cover and simmer 20 minutes.
3. Remove pan from heat. Let stand, covered, 5 minutes or until all liquid is absorbed. Reserve.
4. Heat oil in large non-stick skillet.
5. Sauté onion and celery over moderate heat 3 minutes. Stir in remaining ingredients including reserved cooked rice. Fluff with fork before serving.

Yield: 10 servings
Serving size: ¹/₂ cup

Each serving provides:
Calories: 139
Total fat: 5 g
Saturated fat: less than 1 g

Cholesterol: 0 g
Sodium: 86 mg
Fiber: 1 g
Protein: 3 g
Carbohydrate: 21 g
Potassium: 124 mg

Scallion Rice

4¹/₂ cups rice, cooked in unsalted water
1¹/₂ tsp bouillon granules, unsalted
¹/₄ cup scallions (green onions), chopped

1. Cook rice according to directions on the package.
2. Combine the cooked rice, scallions, and bouillon granules, and mix well.
3. Measure 1-cup portions and serve.

Yield: 5 servings

Serving size: 1 cup

Each serving provides:

Calories: 200

Total fat: 2 g

Saturated fat: 0 g

Cholesterol: 0 g

Sodium: 18 mg

Calcium: 23 mg

Magnesium: 77 mg

Fiber: 6 g

Protein: 5 g

Carbohydrate: 41 g

Potassium: 92 mg

Sunshine Rice

This citrusy rice contains almonds, celery, and onions, but no added salt, for a flavorful low-sodium side dish.

1¹/₂ Tbsp vegetable oil
1¹/₄ cups celery with leaves, finely chopped
1¹/₂ cups onion, finely chopped
1 cup water
¹/₂ cup orange juice
2 Tbsp lemon juice
dash hot sauce
1 cup long-grain white or brown rice, uncooked
¹/₄ cup almonds, slivered

1. Heat oil in medium saucepan. Add celery and onions and sauté until tender, about 10 minutes.
2. Add water, juices, and hot sauce. Bring to a boil. Stir in rice and bring back to a boil. Let stand covered until rice is tender and liquid is absorbed.
3. Stir in slivered almonds. Serve immediately as a side dish for a fish entrée.

Yield: 4 servings	**Cholesterol:** 0 g
Serving size: ¹/₃ cup	**Sodium:** 52 mg
	Fiber: 5 g
Each serving provides:	**Protein:** 7 g
Calories: 276	**Carbohydrate:** 50 g
Total fat: 6 g	**Potassium:** 406 mg
Saturated fat: less than 1 g	

≤ 30 mins   Sides

Vegetables with a Touch of Lemon

This heart-healthy sauce uses lemon juice, herbs, and a small amount of oil.

¹/₂ small head cauliflower, cut into florets
2 cups broccoli, cut into florets
2 Tbsp lemon juice
1 Tbsp olive oil
1 clove garlic, minced
2 tsp fresh parsley, chopped

1. Steam broccoli and cauliflower until tender (about 10 minutes).
2. In a small saucepan, mix the lemon juice, oil, and garlic, and cook over low heat for 2 or 3 minutes.
3. Put the vegetables into a serving dish. Pour the lemon sauce over the vegetables. Garnish with parsley.

Yield: 6 servings
Serving size: ¹/₂ cup

Each serving provides:
Calories: 22
Total fat: 2 g
Saturated fat: less than 1 g
Cholesterol: 0 g

Sodium: 7 mg
Calcium: 10 mg
Iron: less than 1 mg
Fiber: 1 g
Protein: 1 g
Carbohydrate: 2 g
Potassium: 49 mg

New Orleans Red Beans

This vegetarian main dish is cholesterol-free, virtually fat-free, and chock full of vegetables.

1 lb dry red beans
2 qt water
1¹/₂ cups onion, chopped
1 cup celery, chopped
4 bay leaves
1 cup green pepper, chopped
3 Tbsp garlic, chopped
3 Tbsp parsley, chopped
2 tsp dried thyme, crushed
1 tsp salt
1 tsp black pepper

1. Pick through beans to remove bad beans; rinse thoroughly.
2. In a large pot, combine beans, water, onion, celery, and bay leaves. Bring to a boil; reduce heat. Cover and cook over low heat for about 1¹/₂ hours or until beans are tender. Stir. Mash beans against side of pan.
3. Add green pepper, garlic, parsley, thyme, salt, and black pepper. Cook, uncovered, over low heat until creamy, about 30 minutes. Remove bay leaves.
4. Serve with hot cooked brown rice, if desired.

Yield: 8 servings	**Cholesterol:** 0 g
Serving size: 1¹/₄ cups	**Sodium:** 285 mg
	Fiber: 7 g
Each serving provides:	**Protein:** 10 g
Calories: 171	**Carbohydrate:** 32 g
Total fat: less than 1 g	**Potassium:** 665 mg
Saturated fat: less than 1 g	

Sides

New Potato Salad

Onions and spices give this very low-sodium dish plenty of zip.

16 (5 cups) small new potatoes
2 Tbsp olive oil
¹/₄ cup green onions, chopped
¹/₄ tsp black pepper
1 tsp dill weed, dried

1. Thoroughly clean potatoes with vegetable brush and water.
2. Boil potatoes for 20 minutes or until tender.
3. Drain and cool potatoes for 20 minutes.
4. Cut potatoes into fourths and mix with olive oil, onions, and spices.
5. Refrigerate and serve.

Yield: 5 servings
Serving size: 1 cup

Each serving provides:
Calories: 196
Total fat: 6 g
Saturated fat: 1 g

Cholesterol: 0 g
Sodium: 17 mg
Fiber: 4 g
Protein: 4 g
Carbohydrate: 34 g
Potassium: 861 mg

≤ 60 mins   Sides

Smothered Greens with Turkey

Use a small amount of skinless smoked turkey breast instead of fatback to lower the fat content but keep the taste.

3 cups water
$^1/_4$ lb smoked turkey breasts, skinless
1 Tbsp hot pepper, freshly chopped
$^1/_4$ tsp cayenne pepper
$^1/_4$ tsp cloves, ground
2 cloves garlic, crushed
$^1/_2$ tsp thyme
1 stalk scallion, chopped
1 tsp ginger, ground
$^1/_4$ cup onion, chopped
2 lb greens (mustard, turnip, collard, kale, or mixture)

1. Place all ingredients except greens into large saucepan and bring to a boil.
2. Prepare greens by washing thoroughly and removing stems.
3. Tear or slice leaves into bite-size pieces.
4. Add greens to turkey stock.
5. Cook 20-30 minutes until tender.

Yield: 5 servings   Cholesterol: 16 g
Serving size: 1 cup   Sodium: 378 mg
                          Fiber: 4 g
Each serving provides: Protein: 9 g
Calories: 80   Carbohydrate: 9 g
Total fat: 2 g   Potassium: 472 mg
Saturated fat: less than 1 g

Wonderful Stuffed Potatoes

Baked potatoes stuffed with seasoned, low-fat cottage cheese are a lavish low-fat, low-cholesterol, low-sodium treat.

4 medium baking potatoes
3/4 cup cottage cheese, low-fat (1%)
1/4 cup milk, low-fat (1%)
2 Tbsp soft (tub) margarine
1 tsp dill weed
3/4 tsp herb seasoning
4-6 drops hot pepper sauce
2 tsp Parmesan cheese, grated

1. Prick potatoes with fork. Bake at 425° F for 60 minutes or until fork is easily inserted.
2. Cut potatoes in half lengthwise. Carefully scoop out potato, leaving about 1/2 inch of pulp inside shell. Mash pulp in large bowl.
3. Mix in by hand remaining ingredients except Parmesan cheese. Spoon mixture into potato shells.
4. Sprinkle top with 1/4 teaspoon of Parmesan cheese.
5. Place on baking sheet and return to oven. Bake 15-20 minutes or until tops are golden brown.

Yield: 8 servings	**Saturated fat:** 1 g
Serving size: 1/2 potato each	**Cholesterol:** 1 mg
	Sodium: 151 mg
	Fiber: 2 g
Each serving provides:	**Protein:** 5 g
Calories: 113	**Carbohydrate:** 17 g
Total fat: 3 g	**Potassium:** 293 mg

Mousse à la Banana

This creamy dessert is low in saturated fat, cholesterol, and sodium.

2 Tbsp milk, low-fat (1%)
4 tsp sugar
1 tsp vanilla
1 medium banana, cut into quarters
1 cup plain yogurt, low-fat
8 1/4-inch banana slices

1. Place milk, sugar, vanilla, and banana in blender. Process 15 seconds at high speed until smooth.
2. Pour mixture into a small bowl; fold in yogurt. Chill. Spoon into four dessert dishes; garnish each with two banana slices just before serving.

Yield: 4 servings	**Cholesterol:** 4 mg
Serving size: 1/2 cup	**Sodium:** 47 mg
	Fiber: 1 g
Each serving provides:	**Protein:** 1 g
Calories: 94	**Carbohydrate:** 18 g
Total fat: 1 g	**Potassium:** 297 mg
Saturated fat: 1 g	

Desserts

Rainbow Fruit Salad

Good as a side dish or dessert, this salad made from fresh fruit is naturally low in fat, saturated fat, and sodium and is cholesterol-free.

Fruit salad:

1 large mango, peeled and diced
2 cups fresh blueberries
2 bananas, sliced
2 cups fresh strawberries, halved
2 cups seedless grapes
2 nectarines, unpeeled and sliced
1 kiwi fruit, peeled and sliced

Honey orange sauce:

1/3 cup unsweetened orange juice
2 Tbsp lemon juice
1 1/2 Tbsp honey
1/4 tsp ground ginger
dash nutmeg

1. Prepare the fruit.
2. Combine all the ingredients for the sauce and mix.
3. Just before serving, pour honey orange sauce over the fruit.

Yield: 12 servings
Serving size: 4-oz cup

Each serving provides:
Calories: 96
Total fat: 1 g
Saturated fat: less than 1 g

Cholesterol: 0 mg
Sodium: 4 mg
Fiber: 3 g
Protein: 1 g
Carbohydrate: 24 g
Potassium: 302 mg

1-2-3 Peach Cobbler

Cooking oil spray helps to coat the pan with little fat or calories.

¹/₂ tsp cinnamon, ground
1 Tbsp vanilla extract
2 Tbsp cornstarch
1 cup peach nectar
¹/₄ cup pineapple juice or peach juice
2 cans (16 oz) peaches, sliced, packed in juice, and drained (or 1³/₄ lb), fresh
1 Tbsp soft (tub) margarine
1 cup pancake mix, dry
²/₃ cup all-purpose flour
¹/₂ cup sugar
²/₃ cup evaporated milk, fat-free
non-stick cooking oil spray (for baking dish)

Topping:

¹/₂ tsp nutmeg
1 Tbsp brown sugar

1. Combine cinnamon, vanilla, cornstarch, peach nectar, and pineapple or peach juice in a saucepan over medium heat. Stir constantly until mixture thickens and bubbles.
2. Add sliced peaches to mixture.
3. Reduce heat and simmer for 5-10 minutes.
4. In another saucepan, melt margarine and set aside.
5. Lightly spray an 8-inch-square glass dish with cooking oil spray. Pour hot peach mixture into the dish.
6. In another bowl, combine pancake mix, flour, sugar, and melted margarine. Stir in milk.
7. Quickly spoon this mixture over peach mixture.

(continued)

1-2-3 Peach Cobbler (continued)

8. Combine nutmeg and brown sugar. Sprinkle mixture on top of batter.
9. Bake at 400° F for 15-20 minutes or until golden brown.
10. Cool and cut into eight squares.

Yield: 8 servings	**Cholesterol:** less than 1 mg
Serving size: 1 square	**Sodium:** 263 mg
	Fiber: 2 g
Each serving provides:	**Protein:** 4 g
Calories: 271	**Carbohydrate:** 54 g
Total fat: 4 g	**Potassium:** 284 mg
Saturated fat: less than 1 g	

Baked Apple Slices

This recipe provides 1.5 fruit and vegetable servings per person.

2 oranges
2 Tbsp honey
$^1/_4$ tsp ground cinnamon
$^1/_4$ tsp ground cloves
3 Granny Smith apples, peeled, cored, and cut into $^1/_2$-inch slices
5 Tbsp raisins
$^1/_4$ cup chopped walnuts, divided
$^1/_4$ cup vanilla yogurt, low-fat

1. Preheat the oven to 500° F.
2. Grate the zest of one of the oranges and set aside.
3. Squeeze the juice from both oranges into a small bowl. Stir the honey, cinnamon, cloves, and half the zest into the juice.
4. Lay half the apple slices in a glass baking dish. Scatter the raisins and 2 tablespoons of the walnuts on top. Pour on half the juice mixture and top with the remaining apples and juice. Combine the remaining 2 tablespoons of walnuts with the orange zest and scatter over the top.
5. Cover lightly with foil, and bake 30 minutes or until the apples are soft and the juices, bubbly. Serve warm or cold with a dollop of low-fat vanilla yogurt.

Yield: 4 servings	**Total fat:** 6 g
Serving size: ~$1^1/_2$ cups	**Saturated fat:** 1 g
	Carbohydrate: 41 g
Each serving provides:	**Sodium:** 13 mg
Calories: 206	**Fiber:** 4 g

Oatmeal Cookies

³/₄ cup sugar
2 Tbsp margarine
1 egg
¹/₄ cup canned applesauce
2 Tbsp milk, low-fat
1 cup flour
¹/₄ tsp baking soda
¹/₂ tsp ground cinnamon
1 cup + 2 Tbsp quick rolled oats

1. Preheat oven to 350° F and lightly grease cookie sheets.
2. In a large bowl, use an electric mixer on medium speed to mix sugar and margarine. Mix until well blended, about 3 minutes.
3. Slowly add egg; mix on medium speed 1 minute. Gradually add applesauce and milk; mix on medium speed 1 minute. Scrape sides of bowl.
4. In another bowl, combine flour, baking soda, and cinnamon. Slowly add to applesauce mixture; mix on low speed until blended, about 2 minutes. Add oats and blend 30 seconds on low speed. Scrape sides of bowl.
5. Drop by teaspoonfuls onto cookie sheet, about 2 inches apart.
6. Bake until lightly browned, about 13-15 minutes. Remove from baking sheet while still warm. Cool on wire rack.

Yield: 4 servings
Serving size: 2 cookies, plus 4 servings for another snack

Each serving provides:
Calories: 215
Total fat: 4 g
Saturated fat: 1 g
Cholesterol: 27 mg
Sodium: 84 mg

Peach Cake

2¹/₄ cups (29-oz can) canned peaches, light-syrup pack, drained and chopped
¹/₂ cup sugar
1 cup flour
1 egg
1 tsp baking soda
2 Tbsp vegetable oil
1 tsp vanilla
2 Tbsp brown sugar, firmly packed
2 tsp whole milk

1. Preheat oven to 350° F. Lightly grease 8- by 8-inch pan.
2. Spread peaches in baking pan. Mix remaining ingredients, except brown sugar and milk, together in mixing bowl; spread over top of peaches.
3. Bake until toothpick inserted into cake comes out clean, about 30-35 minutes.
4. For topping, combine brown sugar and milk in small bowl. Drizzle mixture on top of cake; return cake to oven, and bake 2-3 minutes.
5. Cut into eight pieces.

Yield: 8 servings
Serving size: about 2- by 2-inch piece

Saturated fat: 1 g
Cholesterol: 27 mg
Sodium: 171 mg

Each serving provides:
Calories: 205
Total fat: 4 g

Peach-Apple Crisp

20 oz canned peaches, light-syrup pack, drained
2 medium apples, tart, peeled and sliced
1/2 tsp vanilla
1/4 tsp ground cinnamon
3/4 cup + 3 Tbsp flour
1/4 cup brown sugar, packed
3 Tbsp soft (tub) margarine

1. Preheat oven to 350° F. Lightly grease 9- by 9- by 2-inch casserole dish.
2. Combine peaches, apples, vanilla, and cinnamon in a bowl. Toss well and spread evenly in greased casserole dish.
3. Combine flour and sugar in small bowl. Cut in margarine with two knives until the mixture resembles coarse meal.
4. Sprinkle flour mixture evenly over fruit.
5. Bake until lightly browned and bubbly, about 20 minutes.

Yield: 4 servings
Serving size: 1/2 cup, plus 4 servings for another meal

Saturated fat: 1 g
Cholesterol: 0 mg
Sodium: 57 mg

Each serving provides:
Calories: 175
Total fat: 5 g

Rice Pudding

Use skim milk instead of whole milk to reduce fat and calories.

| 6 cups water |
| 2 cinnamon sticks |
| 1 cup rice |
| 3 cups milk, fat-free |
| 2/3 cup sugar |
| 1/2 tsp salt |

1. Put the water and cinnamon sticks into a medium saucepan. Bring to a boil.
2. Stir in rice. Cook on low heat for 30 minutes until rice is soft and water has evaporated.
3. Add skim milk, sugar, and salt. Cook for another 15 minutes until it thickens.

Yield: 8 servings
Serving size: 1/2 cup

Each serving provides:
Calories: 372
Total fat: less than 1 g
Saturated fat: less than 1 g
Cholesterol: 3 mg

Sodium: 366 mg
Calcium: 255 mg
Iron: 2 mg
Fiber: 1 g
Protein: 10 g
Carbohydrate: 81 g
Potassium: 363 mg

Sweet Potato Custard

Sweet potatoes and bananas combine to make a flavorful low-fat custard made with evaporated skim milk and no added fat.

1 cup cooked sweet potato, mashed
1/2 cup banana (about 2 small), mashed
1 cup evaporated milk, fat-free
2 Tbsp brown sugar, packed
2 egg yolks, beaten, or 1/3 cup egg substitute
1/2 tsp salt
non-stick cooking spray as needed
1/4 cup raisins
1 Tbsp sugar
1 tsp ground cinnamon

1. In a medium bowl, stir together sweet potato and banana.
2. Add milk, blending well.
3. Add brown sugar, egg yolks, and salt, mixing thoroughly.
4. Spray a 1-quart casserole with non-stick cooking spray. Transfer sweet potato mixture to casserole dish.
5. Combine raisins, sugar, and cinnamon; sprinkle over top of sweet potato mixture.
6. Bake in a preheated 325° F oven for 40-45 minutes or until a knife inserted near center comes out clean.

Yield: 6 servings
Serving size: 1/2 cup

Each serving provides:
Calories: 160
Total fat: 2 g
Saturated fat: less than 1 g
Cholesterol: 72 g*

Sodium: 255 mg
Fiber: 2 g
Protein: 5 g
Carbohydrate: 32 g
Potassium: 488 mg
If egg substitutes are used, cholesterol will be lower.

Winter Crisp

Only 1 tablespoon of margarine is used to make the crumb topping of this tart and tangy fruit dessert that is cholesterol-free and low-sodium.

Filling:

1/2 cup sugar
3 Tbsp all-purpose flour
1 tsp lemon peel, grated
3/4 tsp lemon juice
5 cups apples, unpeeled and sliced
1 cup cranberries

Topping:

2/3 cup rolled oats
1/3 cup brown sugar, packed
1/4 cup whole wheat flour
2 tsp ground cinnamon
1 Tbsp soft (tub) margarine, melted

1. To prepare filling, in a medium bowl combine sugar, flour, and lemon peel; mix well. Add lemon juice, apples, and cranberries; stir to mix. Spoon into a 6-cup baking dish.
2. To prepare topping, in a small bowl, combine oats, brown sugar, flour, and cinnamon. Add melted margarine; stir to mix.
3. Sprinkle topping over filling. Bake in a 375° F oven for approximately 40-50 minutes or until filling is bubbly and top is brown. Serve warm or at room temperature.

(continued)

Variation: Summer Crisp

1. Prepare as directed, substituting 4 cups of fresh or unsweetened frozen (thawed) peaches and 3 cups of fresh or unsweetened frozen (unthawed) blueberries for apples and cranberries. If the peaches are frozen, thaw them completely (do not drain). Do not thaw blueberries before mixing, or they will be crushed.

Yield: 6 servings
Serving size: 1³/₄- by 2-inch piece

Each serving provides:
Calories: 252
Total fat: 2 g

Saturated fat: less than 1 g
Cholesterol: 0 mg
Sodium: 29 mg
Fiber: 5 g
Protein: 3 g
Carbohydrate: 58 g
Potassium: 221 mg

≤ 90 mins   Desserts

Apple Coffee Cake

Apples and raisins provide the moistness, which means less oil can be used in this low-saturated-fat, low-cholesterol, and low-sodium coffee cake.

5 cups tart apples, cored, peeled, and chopped
1 cup sugar
1 cup dark raisins
$^1/_2$ cup pecans, chopped
$^1/_4$ cup vegetable oil
2 tsp vanilla
1 egg, beaten
$2^1/_2$ cups all-purpose flour, sifted
$1^1/_2$ tsp baking soda
2 tsp ground cinnamon

1. Preheat oven to 350° F.
2. Lightly oil a 13- by 9- by 2-inch pan.
3. In a large mixing bowl, combine apples with sugar, raisins, and pecans; mix well. Let stand 30 minutes.
4. Stir in oil, vanilla, and egg. Sift together flour, soda, and cinnamon; stir into apple mixture about $^1/_3$ at a time, just enough to moisten dry ingredients.
5. Turn batter into pan. Bake 35-40 minutes. Cool cake slightly before serving.

Yield: 20 servings
Serving size: $3^1/_2$- by $2^1/_2$-inch piece

Each serving provides:
Calories: 196
Total fat: 8 g
Saturated fat: 1 g
Cholesterol: 11 mg
Sodium: 67 mg
Fiber: 2 g
Protein: 3 g
Carbohydrate: 31 g
Potassium: 136 mg

Frosted Cake

Use fat-free milk and low-fat cream cheese to lower the saturated fat and calories in this special-occasion cake.

Cake:

2¹/₄ cups cake flour
2¹/₄ tsp baking powder
4 Tbsp soft (tub) margarine
1¹/₄ cups sugar
4 eggs
1 tsp vanilla
1 Tbsp orange peel
³/₄ cup milk, fat-free

Icing:

3 oz cream cheese, low-fat
2 Tbsp milk, fat-free
6 Tbsp cocoa
2 cups confectioners sugar, sifted
¹/₂ tsp vanilla extract

1. Preheat the oven to 325° F.
2. Grease with small amount of cooking oil or use non-stick cooking oil spray on a 10-inch round pan (at least 2¹/₂ inches high). Powder pan with flour. Tap out excess flour.
3. Sift together flour and baking powder.
4. In a separate bowl, beat together margarine and sugar until soft and creamy.
5. Beat in eggs, vanilla, and orange peel.
6. Gradually add the flour mixture alternating with the milk, beginning and ending with flour.
7. Pour the mixture into the pan. Bake for 40-45 minutes or until done. Let cake cool for 5-10 minutes before removing from the pan. Let cool completely before icing.

(continued)

Frosted Cake (continued)

Icing:

1. Cream together cream cheese and milk until smooth. Add cocoa. Blend well.
2. Slowly add sugar until icing is smooth. Mix in vanilla.
3. Smooth icing over top and sides of cooled cake.

Yield: 16 servings   **Sodium:** 273 mg
Serving size: 1 slice   **Calcium:** 70 mg
                             Iron: 2 mg
Each serving provides: **Fiber:** 1 g
Calories: 241   **Protein:** 4 g
Total fat: 5 g   **Carbohydrate:** 45 g
Saturated fat: 2 g   **Potassium:** 95 mg
Cholesterol: 57 mg

Web Sites

Nutrition

Dietary Guidelines for Americans 2005
http://www.healthierus.gov/dietaryguidelines/
También se ofrece unas partes en español.

The Dietary Approaches to Stop Hypertension (DASH) Eating Plan
http://www.nhlbi.nih.gov/health/public/heart/hbp/dash/
This Web site contains the DASH Eating Plan and includes information on the research findings that demonstrate its health benefits. The Web site describes the Eating Plan, provides sample 7-day menus and several recipes, and gives helpful tips on how to get started, how to use the DASH Eating Plan if trying to lose weight, how to reduce sodium intake, and how to read and interpret the Nutrition Facts label.

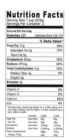

How to Understand and Use the Nutrition Facts Label
http://www.cfsan.fda.gov/~dms/foodlab.html
A useful site that offers easy-to-understand information on Nutrition Facts labels, it offers a sample label with notes on how to tell how much of each listed item is high or low—and what to watch out for. It also gives a consumer-friendly overview of calories, nutrients, and percent Daily Value using additional sample food labels.

Interactive Menu Planner
http://hin.nhlbi.nih.gov/menuplanner/menu.cgi
This site provides an online tool that calculates the servings and calories of your selections from a list of available foods and beverages to make up a meal of specified calories. It also has a link to, among other sites, a Body Mass Index (BMI) calculator and Portion Distortion, which describes the evolution of portion sizes in restaurants.

5 A Day for Better Health

http://5aday.nci.nih.gov/homepage/index_content.html

A site aimed at promoting the healthy consumption of fruits and vegetables among adults, 5 A Day has resources catered to both men and women, including quizzes, scientific evidence, information on serving sizes, and recipes, as well as resources catered to African Americans. The 5 A Day Web site also includes a link to The Color Guide, an informative section on the nutrients associated with fruits and vegetables arranged by color.

Milk Matters

http://www.nichd.nih.gov/milk/

This site provides essential information on the many benefits of milk and calcium. It contains links to up-to-date research on calcium, and campaign-related publications and materials. It also provides a link to the Milk Matters Kids' Page with interactive puzzles and games designed to provide a fun way for kids to learn about the benefits of drinking milk.

También se ofrece en español.

MyPyramid.gov

http://www.mypyramid.gov/

The interactive component of the USDA's new food pyramid, this site allows users to input their age, sex, and amount of daily physical activity to create a personalized food pyramid. The personalized pyramid comes along with recommendations of consumption of specific foods and a meal-tracking worksheet to follow your progress. The site also links to MyPyramid Tracker, a tool that allows users to take an interactive, in-depth assessment of their food intake and physical activity.

Food Safety Fact Sheets

http://www.fsis.usda.gov/fact_sheets/index.asp

This site features helpful food safety fact sheets for safe food handling, meat preparation, poultry preparation, egg product preparation, seasonal food safety, appliances and thermometers, food-borne illness and disease, emergency preparedness, Food Safety and Inspections Service (FSIS) programs and workforce, production and inspection, and food labeling. The site also features Thermy™ temperature charts.

FoodSafety.gov
http://www.foodsafety.gov

FoodSafety.gov is a gateway Web site that provides links to selected government information on food safety. The Consumer Advice section of this site provides extensive access to information about safe food handling and food safety concerns for specific population groups, such as seniors, pregnant women, and children. This site also contains a News and Safety Alerts section with links to product recalls, alerts, and warnings, as well as to other announcements.

Choosing a Safe and Successful Weight Loss Program
http://win.niddk.nih.gov/publications/choosing.htm

This site provides a helpful fact sheet designed to help individuals make informed decisions about weight loss programs. It includes an outline of what safe and effective weight loss programs should include, questions to ask weight loss program providers about everything from cost to contents, and contact information for additional resources.

FirstGov for Consumers: Food
http://www.consumer.gov/food.htm

The food section of FirstGov for consumers is a great resource for consumer information related to fruits and vegetables, seafood, meat and poultry, labeling, nutrition, product recalls, and safety. The site also provides links to several other resources in these areas. Additionally, it offers recipes and an FAQ-format section on consumer advice on food safety, nutrition, and cosmetics with questions ranging from "Why should you not use homemade infant formulas?" to "How will I know if food has been irradiated?" Tambiénse ofrece unas partes en español.

Physical Activity

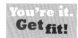

The President's Challenge—You're it. Get fit!
http://www.presidentschallenge.org/

A central component of the President's Council on Physical Fitness and Sports, The President's Challenge—You're it. Get fit!—encourages all Americans to make being active part of their everyday lives. This Web site is the interactive component of that challenge and provides information for kids, teens, adults, and seniors, as well as for teachers and advocates, on how to register, track progress, calculate fitness, and earn awards for meeting goals.

Physical Activity for Everyone
http://www.cdc.gov/nccdphp/dnpa/physical/index.htm

This site provides visitors with an overview of the importance of physical activity and resources to encourage physical activity. The site features a Measuring Physical Activity Intensity section, which includes the Talk Test, target heart rate and estimated maximum heart rate tests, a perceived exertion test, a metabolic equivalent level test, and lists sample activities by intensity level. The site also provides recommendations for physical activity, and a strength training for older adults section, as well as providing links to additional resources.

Recreation.gov
http://www.recreation.gov

A partnership among Federal land management agencies to provide an easy-to-use Web site with information about all federal recreation areas. The site allows you to search for recreation areas by state, by recreational activity, by agency, or by map. It also links visitors to sites where they can make advanced reservations for camp sites and tours, offers recreation maps, and links to weather advisories.

General

HealthierUS.gov
http://www.healthierus.gov

HealthierUS.gov is a Web site supporting the President's HealthierUS initiative focusing on physical fitness, prevention, nutrition, and making healthy choices. It serves as a source of credible, accurate information to help Americans choose to live healthier lives. The site also links to Steps to a HealthierUS (Steps), a bold initiative from the U.S. Department of Health and Human Services that advances President George W. Bush's HealthierUS goal of helping Americans live longer, better, and healthier lives.

healthfinder.gov
http://www.healthfinder.gov/

healthfinder® is a free guide to reliable consumer health information, developed by the U.S. Department of Health and Human Services and other federal agencies. This site links to carefully selected information and Web sites from over 1,700 health-related government agencies and not-for-profit organizations, includes many online checkups, and offers daily health news in English and Spanish.
También se ofrece en español.

SmallStep.gov
http://www.smallstep.gov

In partnership with the Ad Council, SmallStep.gov aims at preventing obesity by encouraging small dietary and physical activity changes in the form of 120 steps, such as Step 5) Drink water before a meal, Step 35) Sit up straight at work, and Step 106) When eating out, ask your server to put half your entrée in a to-go-bag. The site includes the list of steps as well as success stories and tips. Users can sign up for a newsletter with tips, recipes, and more and can create an activity tracker to monitor their progress.
También se ofrece en español.

Nutrition.gov

http://www.nutrition.gov

A service of the National Agricultural Library, U.S. Department of Agriculture, Nutrition.gov is a great resource for up-to-date food and nutrition information. In addition to serving as a gateway to reliable information on nutrition, healthy eating, physical activity, and food safety for consumers, educators, and health professionals, the site offers current food and nutrition news and publications, information on weight management, information on food assistance programs, and also offers grocery-shopping tips.

Audience Specific

You Can!

http://www.aoa.gov/youcan/partners_public/celebration/celebration.asp

This Web site for older adults is to help them make wise food choices and be physically active, strategies that can improve their health and well-being. It provides tips and helps older adults set goals and record progress.

Pick Your Path to Health

http://www.womenshealth.gov/pypth/index.cfm

A site dedicated to the health of women, Pick Your Path to health is an online resource of the Pick Your Path to Health public education campaign to help women take simple and time-sensitive steps to improve their health, and will encourage local communities to promote practical, culturally interesting, and relevant action steps to wellness. The site consists of articles, health calendars, and information on community programs as well as a section on themes and action steps to improve health. The themes and action steps section provides yearly action steps that cater to all women, African American women, Asian and Pacific Islander women, American Indian and Alaska Native women, Latinas, women living in rural areas, women with disabilities, and adolescent girls.

A Parent's Guide to Healthy Eating and Physical Activity
http://www.smallstep.gov/pdf/final_parent_guide_english_%207_27_04.pdf
(Publication)

BAM.gov
http://www.bam.gov
BAM.gov serves as an interactive tool for adolescents that provides up-to-date information and encouragement to increase their level of physical activity and to establish fitness habits that will stay with them for life. The site's Fit4Life section includes fit tips, a personalized fitness and activity calendar, snacking and lunch-packing ideas, activity cards, and a quiz. The site also features Teacher's Corner, which offers suggestions for classroom activities.

VERB™ It's what you do
http://www.cdc.gov/youthcampaign/
An interactive campaign for tweens, VERB™, It's what you do is a national campaign aimed at promoting daily physical activity. VERBnow.com, the site for tweens, is a cool, fun site that provides ideas for physical activity. Kids can also find places to play by selecting a sport and entering their zip code. VERBparents.com, the parent site, features an activity finder, activity ideas, a YMCA locator, an Ask the Expert feature, daily fitness calendars, and message boards to share ideas with other parents. The site also links to SpanishVERB (en español).

Powerful Bones, Powerful Girls
http://www.cdc.gov/powerfulbones/index_content.html
Aimed at promoting healthy bones in adolescent girls, this site features information on calcium and physical activity. The site features the character Carla, who gives tips on meal and snack ideas tailored to adolescent girls, such as ideas for nutrition at the mall and school, on physical activity, and on how to gain information about calcium on food labels. The site also features games, quizzes, a calendar, bone health dictionary, and Web links for further health and fitness information.

We Can! (Ways to Enhance Children's Activity & Nutrition)
http://www.nhlbi.nih.gov
We Can! is a national program designed as a one-stop resource for parents and caregivers interested in practical tools to help children 8 to 13 years old stay at a healthy weight. Tips and fun activities offered to parents, health care providers, and community groups focus on three critical behaviors: improved food choices, increased physical activity, and reduced screen time.

Federal Departments and Agencies

United States Department of Health and Human Services
http://www.hhs.gov/

Centers for Disease Control and Prevention
http://www.cdc.gov/
También se ofrece en español.

Food and Drug Administration
http://www.fda.gov/
También se ofrece en español.

National Institutes of Health
http://www.nih.gov/
También se ofrece en español.

United States Department of Agriculture
http://www.usda.gov/wps/portal/usdahome
También se ofrece en español.

My Money-Saving Tips

It's the food choices made over the long run—day-to-day, week-to-week—that add up to good nutritional health. No one set of menus or recipes, whatever the cost, can satisfy everyone, nor can you always eat as planned. Being flexible is part of making healthy eating fit into your lifestyle and budget.

 ## Before Going to the Store

- *Eat something healthy.* Don't shop hungry.
- *In the kitchen, make a list of meal ideas* for the coming week. Keep in mind the days you'll have time to cook from scratch and the days you'll be pressed for time. Then, make a grocery list and stick to it.
- *Review store ads, clip coupons, and organize* them at home.

 ## At the Grocery Store

- *Sign up for your grocer's bonus/discount card* for additional savings.
- *Try store brands.* The most costly brands are often placed at eye-level. Store brands that may be cheaper and just as good are often placed higher or lower on the grocery shelves.
- *Look for the unit price to compare similar foods.* It tells you the cost per ounce, pound, or pint, so you'll know which brand or size is the best buy. Most stores show the unit price on a shelf sticker just below the product.
- *Buy in-season fruits and vegetables.* Use local farmers' markets when possible— the foods are fresher and tend to cost less.
- *Purchase canned (in water or in their own juice, not heavy syrup) and frozen fruits and vegetables.* They're healthy, too, and will last longer.
- *Buy milk (fat-free or low-fat) in large containers* (gallon or 1/2 gallon) that generally cost less than milk in quart containers. Milk sold at "24-hour" convenience stores usually costs more than that sold at supermarket food stores. (Non-fat dry milk is the least expensive way to go.)
- *The whole may be cheaper than the parts*—buy a whole chicken and cut it into pieces at home instead of buying pre-cut chicken (breasts, legs, and wings) that may be more expensive.

- *Stock up on sale items* you can use in a timely manner. Buy in bulk for quality and value, but serve healthy portions.
- *Use your food budget wisely.* For the price of a large bag of chips and a box of cookies, you can buy a lot of apples, bananas, carrots, potatoes, peppers, and other healthier foods.

 For Later at Home

- *Assemble healthy snacks at home* in small baggies using foods such as nuts and seeds, low-fat cheese, and fresh veggies and fruits, rather than buying less healthy and more expensive prepackaged and processed snacks.
- *Do "batch cooking"* when the food budget and time allow. Cook a large amount of spaghetti sauce, divide it into family-size portions, and freeze them promptly for meals later in the month.
- *Take advantage of planned leftovers* to cut preparation time and save food dollars. For example, prepare a roast, serve half of it, and freeze the remaining half to use later with vegetables for a quick soup or in other dishes.

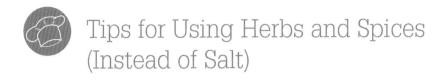

Tips for Using Herbs and Spices (Instead of Salt)

Basil: Use in soups, salads, vegetables, fish, and meats.

Cinnamon: Use in salads, vegetables, breads, and snacks.

Chili Powder: Use in soups, salads, vegetables, and fish.

Cloves: Use in soups, salads, and vegetables.

Dill Weed and Dill Seed: Use in fish, soups, salads, and vegetables.

Ginger: Use in soups, salads, vegetables, and meats.

Marjoram: Use in soups, salads, vegetables, beef, fish, and chicken.

Nutmeg: Use in vegetables, meats, and snacks.

Oregano: Use in soups, salads, vegetables, meats, and chicken.

Parsley: Use in salads, vegetables, fish, and meats.

Rosemary: Use in salads, vegetables, fish, and meats.

Sage: Use in soups, salads, vegetables, meats, and chicken.

Thyme: Use in salads, vegetables, fish, and chicken.

Note: To start, use small amounts of these herbs and spices to see whether you like them.

Source: http://hin.nhlbi.nih.gov/nhbpep_kit/herbs.htm

Play It Safe With Food

Becoming a Healthier You means knowing how to prepare, handle, and store food safely. Follow these tips to keep you and your family safe:

- Clean hands, food-contact surfaces, fruits, and vegetables. To avoid spreading bacteria to other foods, meat and poultry should not be washed or rinsed. (Splashing water while rinsing meat and poultry may cause cross-contamination.)
- Separate raw, cooked, and ready-to-eat foods while shopping, preparing, or storing.
- Cook meat, poultry, and fish to safe internal temperatures to kill microorganisms.
- Chill (refrigerate) perishable foods promptly and thaw/defrost foods properly.

> **The "Right and Left" About Washing Hands**
>
> Wet hands (both of them!); apply soap; rub hands vigorously together— 20 seconds (the time it takes to sing "Happy Birthday" twice); rinse hands thoroughly under clean, running warm water; dry hands completely; best to do with a clean disposable or cloth towel.

Reminder

For infants and young children, pregnant women, older adults, and those with weakened immune systems:
- Do not eat or drink raw (unpasteurized) milk or any product made from unpasteurized milk, raw or partially cooked eggs or food containing raw eggs, raw or undercooked meat and poultry, unpasteurized juices, and raw sprouts.

Pregnant women, older adults, and those with weakened immune systems:
- Only eat certain deli meats and frankfurters that have been reheated to steaming hot.

Temperature Rules!

For safe cooking and handling of food—know that bacteria multiply rapidly between 40°F and 140°F, doubling in number in as little as 20 minutes. To keep food out of this danger zone, keep cold food cold and hot food hot. Keep food cold in the refrigerator, in coolers, or on the service line on ice. Set your refrigerator no higher than 40°F and the freezer at 0°F. Keep food hot in the oven, in heated chafing dishes, or in preheated steam tables, warming trays, and/or slow cookers. Use a clean thermometer that measures the internal temperature of cooked food to make sure meats, poultry, and casseroles are cooked to the temperatures as indicated in the figure.

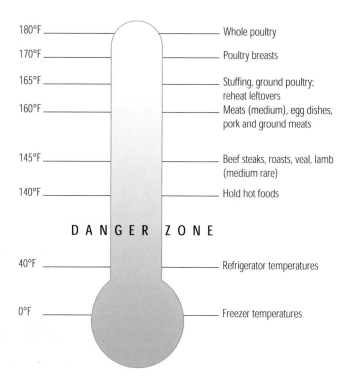

180°F — Whole poultry

170°F — Poultry breasts

165°F — Stuffing, ground poultry; reheat leftovers

160°F — Meats (medium), egg dishes, pork and ground meats

145°F — Beef steaks, roasts, veal, lamb (medium rare)

140°F — Hold hot foods

D A N G E R Z O N E

40°F — Refrigerator temperatures

0°F — Freezer temperatures

Part V

Dietary Guidelines for Americans 2005

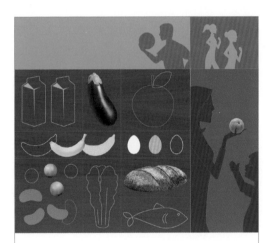

Dietary Guidelines
for Americans
2005

U.S. Department of Health and Human Services
U.S. Department of Agriculture
www.healthierus.gov/dietaryguidelines

Executive Summary

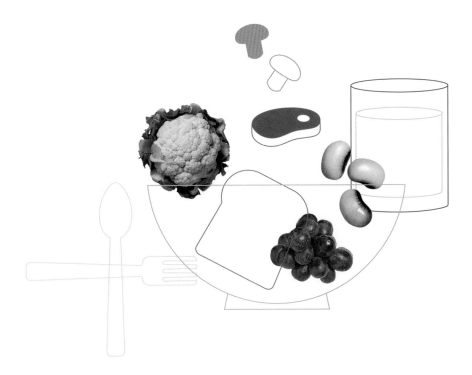

The *Dietary Guidelines for Americans [Dietary Guidelines]* provides science-based advice to promote health and to reduce risk for major chronic diseases through diet and physical activity. Major causes of morbidity and mortality in the United States are related to poor diet and a sedentary lifestyle. Some specific diseases linked to poor diet and physical inactivity include cardiovascular disease, type 2 diabetes, hypertension, osteoporosis, and certain cancers. Furthermore, poor diet and physical inactivity, resulting in an energy imbalance (more calories consumed than expended), are the most important factors contributing to the increase in overweight and obesity in this country. Combined with physical activity, following a diet that does not provide excess calories according to the recommendations in this document should enhance the health of most individuals.

An important component of each 5-year revision of the *Dietary Guidelines* is the analysis of new scientific information by the Dietary Guidelines Advisory Committee (DGAC) appointed by the Secretaries of the U.S. Department of Health and Human

Services (HHS) and the U.S. Department of Agriculture (USDA). This analysis, published in the DGAC Report (http://www.health.gov/dietaryguidelines/dga2005/ report/), is the primary resource for development of the report on the Guidelines by the Departments. The *Dietary Guidelines* and the report of the DGAC differ in scope and purpose compared to reports for previous versions of the *Guidelines*. The 2005 DGAC report is a detailed scientific analysis. The scientific report was used to develop the *Dietary Guidelines* jointly between the two Departments and forms the basis of recommendations that will be used by USDA and HHS for program and policy development. Thus it is a publication oriented toward policymakers, nutrition educators, nutritionists, and healthcare providers rather than to the general public, as with previous versions of the *Dietary Guidelines*, and contains more technical information.

The intent of the *Dietary Guidelines* is to summarize and synthesize knowledge regarding individual nutrients and food components into recommendations for a pattern of eating that can be adopted by the public. In this publication, Key Recommendations are grouped under nine inter-related focus areas. The recommendations are based on the preponderance of scientific evidence for lowering risk of chronic disease and promoting health. It is important to remember that these are integrated messages that should be implemented as a whole. Taken together, they encourage most Americans to eat fewer calories, be more active, and make wiser food choices.

A basic premise of the *Dietary Guidelines* is that nutrient needs should be met primarily through consuming foods. Foods provide an array of nutrients and other compounds that may have beneficial effects on health. In certain cases, fortified foods and dietary supplements may be useful sources of one or more nutrients that otherwise might be consumed in less than recommended amounts. However, dietary supplements, while recommended in some cases, cannot replace a healthful diet.

Two examples of eating patterns that exemplify the *Dietary Guidelines* are the USDA Food Guide (http:// www.usda.gov/cnpp/pyramid.html) and the DASH (Dietary Approaches to Stop Hypertension) Eating Plan.[1] Both of these eating patterns are designed to integrate dietary recommendations into a healthy way to eat for most individuals. These eating patterns are not weight loss diets, but rather illustrative examples of how to eat in accordance with the *Dietary Guidelines*. Both eating patterns are constructed across a range of calorie levels to meet the needs of various age and gender groups. For the USDA Food Guide, nutrient content estimates for each food group and subgroup are based on population-weighted food intakes. Nutrient content

[1] NIH Publication No. 03-4082, Facts about the DASH Eating Plan, United States Department of Health and Human Services, National Institutes of Health, National Heart, Lung, and Blood Institute, Karanja NM et al. *Journal of the American Dietetic Association (JADA)* 8:S19-27, 1999. http://www.nhlbi.nih.gov/health/public/heart/hbp/dash/.

estimates for the DASH Eating Plan are based on selected foods chosen for a sample 7-day menu. While originally developed to study the effects of an eating pattern on the prevention and treatment of hypertension, DASH is one example of a balanced eating plan consistent with the 2005 *Dietary Guidelines*.

Taken together, [the *Dietary Guidelines*] encourage most Americans to eat fewer calories, be more active, and make wiser food choices.

Throughout most of this publication, examples use a 2,000-calorie level as a reference for consistency with the Nutrition Facts Panel. Although this level is used as a reference, recommended calorie intake will differ for individuals based on age, gender, and activity level. At each calorie level, individuals who eat nutrient-dense foods may be able to meet their recommended nutrient intake without consuming their full calorie allotment. The remaining calories—the *discretionary calorie allowance*— allow individuals flexibility to consume some foods and beverages that may contain added fats, added sugars, and alcohol.

The recommendations in the *Dietary Guidelines* are for Americans over 2 years of age. It is important to incorporate the food preferences of different racial/ethnic groups, vegetarians, and other groups when planning diets and developing educational programs and materials. The USDA Food Guide and the DASH Eating Plan are flexible enough to accommodate a range of food preferences and cuisines.

The *Dietary Guidelines* is intended primarily for use by policymakers, healthcare providers, nutritionists, and nutrition educators. The information in the *Dietary Guidelines* is useful for the development of educational materials and aids policymakers in designing and implementing nutrition-related programs, including federal food, nutrition education, and information programs. In addition, this publication has the potential to provide authoritative statements as provided for in the Food and Drug Administration Modernization Act (FDAMA). Because the *Dietary Guidelines* contains discussions where the science is emerging, only statements included in the Executive Summary and the sections titled "Key Recommendations," which reflect the preponderance of scientific evidence, can be used for identification of authoritative statements. The recommendations are inter-related and mutually dependent; thus the statements in this document should be used together in the context of planning an overall healthful diet. However, even following just some of the recommendations can have health benefits.

The following is a listing of the *Dietary Guidelines* by topic.

ADEQUATE NUTRIENTS WITHIN CALORIE NEEDS
Key Recommendations
- Consume a variety of nutrient-dense foods and beverages within and among the basic food groups while choosing foods that limit the intake of saturated and *trans* fats, cholesterol, added sugars, salt, and alcohol.
- Meet recommended intakes within energy needs by adopting a balanced eating pattern, such as the USDA Food Guide or the DASH Eating Plan.

Key Recommendations for Specific Population Groups
- *People over age 50.* Consume vitamin B_{12} in its crystalline form (i.e., fortified foods or supplements).
- *Women of childbearing age who may become pregnant.* Eat foods high in heme-iron and/or consume iron-rich plant foods or iron-fortified foods with an enhancer of iron absorption, such as vitamin C-rich foods.
- *Women of childbearing age who may become pregnant and those in the first trimester of pregnancy.* Consume adequate synthetic folic acid daily (from fortified foods or supplements) in addition to food forms of folate from a varied diet.
- *Older adults, people with dark skin, and people exposed to insufficient ultraviolet band radiation (i.e., sunlight).* Consume extra vitamin D from vitamin D-fortified foods and/or supplements.

WEIGHT MANAGEMENT
Key Recommendations
- To maintain body weight in a healthy range, balance calories from foods and beverages with calories expended.
- To prevent gradual weight gain over time, make small decreases in food and beverage calories and increase physical activity.

Key Recommendations for Specific Population Groups

- *Those who need to lose weight.* Aim for a slow, steady weight loss by decreasing calorie intake while maintaining an adequate nutrient intake and increasing physical activity.
- *Overweight children.* Reduce the rate of body weight gain while allowing growth and development. Consult a healthcare provider before placing a child on a weight-reduction diet.
- *Pregnant women.* Ensure appropriate weight gain as specified by a healthcare provider.
- *Breastfeeding women.* Moderate weight reduction is safe and does not compromise weight gain of the nursing infant.
- *Overweight adults and overweight children with chronic diseases and/or on medication.* Consult a healthcare provider about weight loss strategies prior to starting a weight-reduction program to ensure appropriate management of other health conditions.

PHYSICAL ACTIVITY

Key Recommendations

- Engage in regular physical activity and reduce sedentary activities to promote health, psychological well-being, and a healthy body weight.
  - To reduce the risk of chronic disease in adulthood: Engage in at least 30 minutes of moderate-intensity physical activity, above usual activity, at work or home on most days of the week.
  - For most people, greater health benefits can be obtained by engaging in physical activity of more vigorous intensity or longer duration.
  - To help manage body weight and prevent gradual, unhealthy body weight gain in adulthood: Engage in approximately 60 minutes of moderate- to vigorous-intensity activity on most days of the week while not exceeding caloric intake requirements.
  - To sustain weight loss in adulthood: Participate in at least 60 to 90 minutes of daily moderate-intensity physical activity while not exceeding caloric intake requirements. Some people may need to consult with a healthcare provider before participating in this level of activity.
- Achieve physical fitness by including cardiovascular conditioning, stretching exercises for flexibility, and resistance exercises or calisthenics for muscle strength and endurance.

Key Recommendations for Specific Population Groups

- *Children and adolescents.* Engage in at least 60 minutes of physical activity on most, preferably all, days of the week.
- *Pregnant women.* In the absence of medical or obstetric complications, incorporate 30 minutes or more of moderate-intensity physical activity on most, if not all, days of the week. Avoid activities with a high risk of falling or abdominal trauma.
- *Breastfeeding women.* Be aware that neither acute nor regular exercise adversely affects the mother's ability to successfully breastfeed.
- *Older adults.* Participate in regular physical activity to reduce functional declines associated with aging and to achieve the other benefits of physical activity identified for all adults.

FOOD GROUPS TO ENCOURAGE
Key Recommendations

- Consume a sufficient amount of fruits and vegetables while staying within energy needs. Two cups of fruit and 2½ cups of vegetables per day are recommended for a reference 2,000-calorie intake, with higher or lower amounts depending on the calorie level.
- Choose a variety of fruits and vegetables each day. In particular, select from all five vegetable subgroups (dark green, orange, legumes, starchy vegetables, and other vegetables) several times a week.
- Consume 3 or more ounce-equivalents of whole-grain products per day, with the rest of the recommended grains coming from enriched or whole-grain products. In general, at least half the grains should come from whole grains.
- Consume 3 cups per day of fat-free or low-fat milk or equivalent milk products.

Key Recommendations for Specific Population Groups

- *Children and adolescents.* Consume whole-grain products often; at least half the grains should be whole grains. Children 2 to 8 years should consume 2 cups per day of fat-free or low-fat milk or equivalent milk products. Children 9 years of age and older should consume 3 cups per day of fat-free or low-fat milk or equivalent milk products.

FATS
Key Recommendations

- Consume less than 10 percent of calories from saturated fatty acids and less than 300 mg/day of cholesterol, and keep *trans* fatty acid consumption as low as possible.
- Keep total fat intake between 20 to 35 percent of calories, with most fats coming from sources of polyunsaturated and monounsaturated fatty acids, such as fish, nuts, and vegetable oils.

- When selecting and preparing meat, poultry, dry beans, and milk or milk products, make choices that are lean, low-fat, or fat-free.
- Limit intake of fats and oils high in saturated and/or *trans* fatty acids, and choose products low in such fats and oils.

Key Recommendations for Specific Population Groups

- *Children and adolescents.* Keep total fat intake between 30 to 35 percent of calories for children 2 to 3 years of age and between 25 to 35 percent of calories for children and adolescents 4 to 18 years of age, with most fats coming from sources of polyunsaturated and monounsaturated fatty acids, such as fish, nuts, and vegetable oils.

CARBOHYDRATES
Key Recommendations

- Choose fiber-rich fruits, vegetables, and whole grains often.
- Choose and prepare foods and beverages with little added sugars or caloric sweeteners, such as amounts suggested by the USDA Food Guide and the DASH Eating Plan.
- Reduce the incidence of dental caries by practicing good oral hygiene and consuming sugar- and starch-containing foods and beverages less frequently.

SODIUM AND POTASSIUM
Key Recommendations

- Consume less than 2,300 mg (approximately 1 tsp of salt) of sodium per day.
- Choose and prepare foods with little salt. At the same time, consume potassium-rich foods, such as fruits and vegetables.

Key Recommendations for Specific Population Groups

- *Individuals with hypertension, blacks, and middle-aged and older adults.* Aim to consume no more than 1,500 mg of sodium per day, and meet the potassium recommendation (4,700 mg/day) with food.

ALCOHOLIC BEVERAGES
Key Recommendations

- Those who choose to drink alcoholic beverages should do so sensibly and in moderation—defined as the consumption of up to one drink per day for women and up to two drinks per day for men.
- Alcoholic beverages should not be consumed by some individuals, including those who cannot restrict their alcohol intake, women of childbearing age who

may become pregnant, pregnant and lactating women, children and adolescents, individuals taking medications that can interact with alcohol, and those with specific medical conditions.

- Alcoholic beverages should be avoided by individuals engaging in activities that require attention, skill, or coordination, such as driving or operating machinery.

FOOD SAFETY

Key Recommendations

- To avoid microbial foodborne illness:
  - Clean hands, food contact surfaces, and fruits and vegetables. Meat and poultry should *not* be washed or rinsed.
  - Separate raw, cooked, and ready-to-eat foods while shopping, preparing, or storing foods.
  - Cook foods to a safe temperature to kill microorganisms.
  - Chill (refrigerate) perishable food promptly and defrost foods properly.
  - Avoid raw (unpasteurized) milk or any products made from unpasteurized milk, raw or partially cooked eggs or foods containing raw eggs, raw or under-cooked meat and poultry, unpasteurized juices, and raw sprouts.

Key Recommendations for Specific Population Groups

- *Infants and young children, pregnant women, older adults, and those who are immunocompromised.* Do not eat or drink raw (unpasteurized) milk or any products made from unpasteurized milk, raw or partially cooked eggs or foods containing raw eggs, raw or undercooked meat and poultry, raw or undercooked fish or shell-fish, unpasteurized juices, and raw sprouts.
- *Pregnant women, older adults, and those who are immunocompromised.* Only eat certain deli meats and frankfurters that have been reheated to steaming hot.

Background and Purpose of the *Dietary Guidelines for Americans*

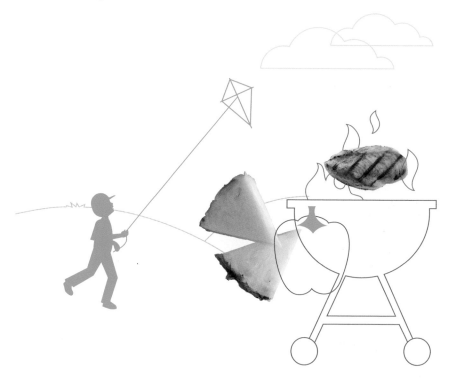

The *Dietary Guidelines for Americans [Dietary Guidelines]*, first published in 1980, provides science-based advice to promote health and to reduce risk for chronic diseases through diet and physical activity. The recommendations contained within the *Dietary Guidelines* are targeted to the general public over 2 years of age who are living in the United States. Because of its focus on health promotion and risk reduction, the *Dietary Guidelines* form the basis of federal food, nutrition education, and information programs.

By law (Public Law 101-445, Title III, 7 U.S.C. 5301 et seq.), the *Dietary Guidelines* is reviewed, updated if necessary, and published every 5 years. The process to create the *Dietary Guidelines* is a joint effort of the U.S. Department of Health and Human Services (HHS) and the U.S. Department of Agriculture (USDA) and has evolved to include three stages.

In the first stage, an external scientific Advisory Committee appointed by the two Departments conducted an analysis of new scientific information and prepared a report summarizing its findings.[2] The Advisory Committee's report was made available to the public and Government agencies for comment. The Committee's analysis was the primary resource for development of the *Dietary Guidelines* by the Departments. A significant amount of the new scientific information used by the Dietary Guidelines Advisory Committee (DGAC) was based on the Dietary Reference Intake (DRI) reports published since 2000 by the Institute of Medicine (IOM), in particular the macronutrient report and the fluid and electrolyte report.

During the second stage, the Departments jointly developed Key Recommendations based on the Advisory Committee's report and public and agency comments. The *Dietary Guidelines* details these science-based policy recommendations. Finally, in the third stage, the two Departments developed messages communicating the *Dietary Guidelines* to the general public.

Because of the three-part process used to develop and communicate the 2005 *Dietary Guidelines*, this publication and the report of the DGAC differ in scope and purpose compared to reports for previous versions of the *Guidelines*. The 2005 DGAC report is a detailed scientific analysis that identifies key issues such as energy balance, the consequences of a sedentary lifestyle, and the need to emphasize certain food choices to address nutrition issues for the American public. The scientific report was used to develop the *Dietary Guidelines* jointly between the two Departments, and this publication forms the basis of recommendations that will be used by USDA and HHS for program and policy development. Thus it is a publication oriented toward policymakers, nutrition educators, nutritionists and healthcare providers rather than to the general public, as with previous versions of the *Dietary Guidelines*, and contains more technical information.

New sections in the *Dietary Guidelines*, consistent with its use for program development, are a glossary of terms (page 340) and appendixes (pages 319 to 339) with detailed information about the USDA Food Guide and the Dietary Approaches to Stop Hypertension (DASH) Eating Plan as well as tables listing sources of some nutrients. Consumer messages have been developed to educate the public about the Key Recommendations in the *Dietary Guidelines* and will be used in materials targeted for consumers separate from this publication. In organizing the *Dietary Guidelines*

---

[2] For more information about the process, summary data, and the resources used by the Advisory Committee, see the 2005 Dietary Guidelines Advisory Committee Report (2005 DGAC Report) at http://www.health.gov/dietaryguidelines.

for the Departments, titles characterize the topic of each section, and the *Dietary Guidelines* itself is presented as an integrated set of Key Recommendations in each topic area.

These Key Recommendations are based on a preponderance of the scientific evidence of nutritional factors that are important for lowering risk of chronic disease and promoting health. To optimize the beneficial impact of these recommendations on health, the *Guidelines* should be implemented in their entirety.

IMPORTANCE OF THE *DIETARY GUIDELINES* FOR HEALTH PROMOTION AND DISEASE PREVENTION

Good nutrition is vital to good health and is absolutely essential for the healthy growth and development of children and adolescents. Major causes of morbidity and mortality in the United States are related to poor diet and a sedentary lifestyle. Specific diseases and conditions linked to poor diet include cardiovascular disease, hypertension, dyslipidemia, type 2 diabetes, overweight and obesity, osteoporosis, constipation, diverticular disease, iron deficiency anemia, oral disease, malnutrition, and some cancers. Lack of physical activity has been associated with cardiovascular disease, hypertension, overweight and obesity, osteoporosis, diabetes, and certain cancers. Furthermore, muscle strengthening and improving balance can reduce falls and increase functional status among older adults. Together with physical activity, a high-quality diet that does not provide excess calories should enhance the health of most individuals.

Poor diet and physical inactivity, resulting in an energy imbalance (more calories consumed than expended), are the most important factors contributing to the increase in overweight and obesity in this country. Moreover, overweight and obesity are major risk factors for certain chronic diseases such as diabetes. In 1999–2002, 65 percent of U.S. adults were overweight, an increase from 56 percent in 1988–1994. Data from 1999–2002 also showed that 30 percent of adults were obese, an increase from 23 percent in an earlier survey. Dramatic increases in the prevalence of overweight have occurred in children and adolescents of both sexes, with approximately 16 percent of children and adolescents aged 6 to 19 years considered to be overweight (1999–2002).[3] In order to reverse this trend, many Americans need to consume fewer calories, be more active, and make wiser choices within and among food groups. The *Dietary Guidelines* provides a framework to promote healthier lifestyles (see Weight Management, pages 269 to 275).

---

[3] Hedley AA, Ogden CL, Johnson CL, Carroll MD, Curtin LR, Flegal KM. Prevalence of overweight and obesity among U.S. children, adolescents, and adults, 1999-2002. *Journal of the American Medical Association (JAMA)* 291(23):2847-2850, 2004.

Given the importance of a balanced diet to health, the intent of the *Dietary Guidelines* is to summarize and synthesize knowledge regarding individual nutrients and food components into recommendations for an overall pattern of eating that can be adopted by the general public. These patterns are exemplified by the USDA Food Guide and the DASH Eating Plan (see Adequate Nutrients Within Calorie Needs, pages 320 to 327). The *Dietary Guidelines* is applicable to the food preferences of different racial/ethnic groups, vegetarians, and other groups. This concept of balanced eating patterns should be utilized in planning diets for various population groups.

There is a growing body of evidence which demonstrates that following a diet that complies with the *Dietary Guidelines* may reduce the risk of chronic disease. Recently, it was reported that dietary patterns consistent with recommended dietary guidance were associated with a lower risk of mortality among individuals age 45 years and older in the United States.[4] The authors of the study estimated that about 16 percent and 9 percent of mortality from any cause in men and women, respectively, could be eliminated by the adoption of desirable dietary behaviors. Currently, adherence to the *Dietary Guidelines* is low among the U.S. population. Data from USDA illustrate the degree of change in the overall dietary pattern of Americans needed to be consistent with a food pattern encouraged by the *Dietary Guidelines* (fig. 1, page 256).

A basic premise of the *Dietary Guidelines* is that nutrient needs should be met primarily through consuming foods. Foods provide an array of nutrients (as well as phytochemicals, antioxidants, etc.) and other compounds that may have beneficial effects on health. In some cases, fortified foods may be useful sources of one or more nutrients that otherwise might be consumed in less than recommended amounts. Supplements may be useful when they fill a specific identified nutrient gap that cannot or is not otherwise being met by the individual's intake of food. Nutrient supplements cannot replace a healthful diet. Individuals who are already consuming the recommended amount of a nutrient in food will not achieve any additional health benefit if they also take the nutrient as a supplement. In fact, in some cases, supplements and fortified foods may cause intakes to exceed the safe levels of nutrients. Another important premise of the *Dietary Guidelines* is that foods should be prepared and handled in such a way that reduces risk of foodborne illness.

[4] Kant AK, Graubard BI, Schatzkin A. Dietary patterns predict mortality in a national cohort: The national health interview surveys, 1987 and 1992. *Journal of Nutrition (J Nutr)* 134:1793-1799, 2004.

USES OF THE *DIETARY GUIDELINES*

The *Dietary Guidelines* is intended primarily for use by policymakers, healthcare providers, nutritionists, and nutrition educators. While the *Dietary Guidelines* was developed for healthy Americans 2 years of age and older, where appropriate, the needs of specific population groups have been addressed. In addition, other individuals may find this report helpful in making healthful choices. As noted previously, the recommendations contained within the *Dietary Guidelines* will aid the public in reducing their risk for obesity and chronic disease. Specific uses of the *Dietary Guidelines* include:

Development of Educational Materials and Communications.

The information in the *Dietary Guidelines* is useful for the development of educational materials. For example, the federal dietary guidance-related publications are required by law to be based on the *Dietary Guidelines*. In addition, this publication will guide the development of messages to communicate the *Dietary Guidelines* to the public. Finally, the USDA Food Guide, the food label, and Nutrition Facts Panel provide information that is useful for implementing the key recommendations in the *Dietary Guidelines* and should be integrated into educational and communication messages.

Development of Nutrition-Related Programs.

The *Dietary Guidelines* aids policymakers in designing and implementing nutrition-related programs. The Federal Government bases its nutrition programs, such as the National Child Nutrition Programs or the Elderly Nutrition Program, on the *Dietary Guidelines*.

Development of Authoritative Statements.

The *Dietary Guidelines* has the potential to provide authoritative statements as provided for in the Food and Drug Administration Modernization Act (FDAMA). Because the recommendations are interrelated and mutually dependent, the statements in this publication should be used together in the context of an overall healthful diet. Likewise, because the *Dietary Guidelines* contains discussions about emerging science, only statements included in the Executive Summary and the highlighted boxes entitled "Key Recommendations," which reflect the preponderance of scientific evidence, can be used for identification of authoritative statements.

FIGURE 1. Percent Increase or Decrease From Current Consumption (Zero Line) to Recommended Intakes[a,b]

A graphical depiction of the degree of change in average daily food consumption by Americans that would be needed to be consistent with the food patterns encouraged by the *Dietary Guidelines for Americans*. The zero line represents average consumption levels from each food group or subgroup by females 31 to 50 years of age and males 31 to 50 years of age. Bars above the zero line represent recommended increases in food group consumption, while bars below the line represent recommended decreases.

Food Groups and Oils

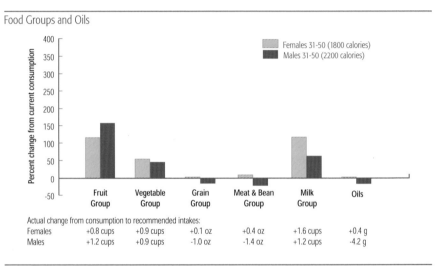

Actual change from consumption to recommended intakes:

	Fruit Group	Vegetable Group	Grain Group	Meat & Bean Group	Milk Group	Oils
Females	+0.8 cups	+0.9 cups	+0.1 oz	+0.4 oz	+1.6 cups	+0.4 g
Males	+1.2 cups	+0.9 cups	-1.0 oz	-1.4 oz	+1.2 cups	-4.2 g

Subgroups, Solid Fats, and Added Sugars

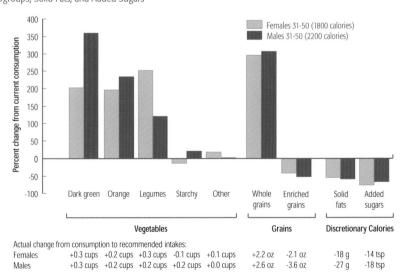

Actual change from consumption to recommended intakes:

	Dark green	Orange	Legumes	Starchy	Other	Whole grains	Enriched grains	Solid fats	Added sugars
Females	+0.3 cups	+0.2 cups	+0.3 cups	-0.1 cups	+0.1 cups	+2.2 oz	-2.1 oz	-18 g	-14 tsp
Males	+0.3 cups	+0.2 cups	+0.2 cups	+0.2 cups	+0.0 cups	+2.6 oz	-3.6 oz	-27 g	-18 tsp

[a] USDA Food Guide in comparison to National Health and Nutrition Examination Survey 2001-2002 consumption data.

[b] Increases in amounts of some food groups are offset by decreases in amounts of solid fats (i.e., saturated and *trans* fats) and added sugars so that total calorie intake is at the recommended level.

Adequate Nutrients Within Calorie Needs

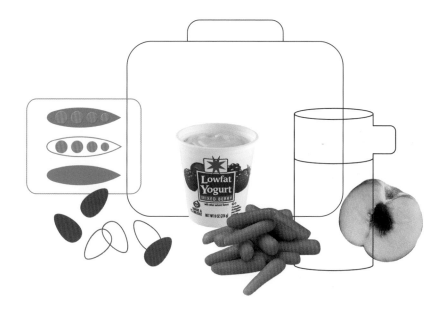

OVERVIEW

Many Americans consume more calories than they need without meeting recommended intakes for a number of nutrients. This circumstance means that most people need to choose meals and snacks that are high in nutrients but low to moderate in energy content; that is, meeting nutrient recommendations must go hand in hand with keeping calories under control. Doing so offers important benefits—normal growth and development of children, health promotion for people of all ages, and reduction of risk for a number of chronic diseases that are major public health problems.

Based on dietary intake data or evidence of public health problems, intake levels of the following nutrients may be of concern for:
- Adults: calcium, potassium, fiber, magnesium, and vitamins A (as carotenoids), C, and E,
- Children and adolescents: calcium, potassium, fiber, magnesium, and vitamin E,

- Specific population groups (see page 259): vitamin B_{12}, iron, folic acid, and vitamins E and D.

At the same time, in general, Americans consume too many calories and too much saturated and *trans* fats, cholesterol, added sugars, and salt.

DISCUSSION

Meeting Recommended Intakes Within Energy Needs

A basic premise of the *Dietary Guidelines* is that food guidance should recommend diets that will provide all the nutrients needed for growth and health. To this end, food guidance should encourage individuals to achieve the most recent nutrient intake recommendations of the Institute of Medicine, referred to collectively as the Dietary Reference Intakes (DRIs). Tables of the DRIs are provided at http://www.iom.edu/Object.File/Master/21/372/0.pdf.

An additional premise of the *Dietary Guidelines* is that the nutrients consumed should come primarily from foods. Foods contain not only the vitamins and minerals that are often found in supplements, but also hundreds of naturally occurring substances, including carotenoids, flavonoids and isoflavones, and protease inhibitors that may protect against chronic health conditions. There are instances when fortified foods may be advantageous, as identified on the pages that follow. These include providing additional sources of certain nutrients that might otherwise be present only in low amounts in some food sources, providing nutrients in highly bioavailable forms, and where the fortification addresses a documented public health need.

Two examples of eating patterns that exemplify the *Dietary Guidelines* are the DASH Eating Plan and the USDA Food Guide. These two similar eating patterns are designed to integrate dietary recommendations into a healthy way to eat and are used in the *Dietary Guidelines* to provide examples of how nutrient-focused recommendations can be expressed in terms of food choices. Both the USDA Food Guide and the DASH Eating Plan differ in important ways from common food consumption patterns in the United States. In general, they include:

- *More* dark green vegetables, orange vegetables, legumes, fruits, whole grains, and low-fat milk and milk products.
- *Less* refined grains, total fats (especially cholesterol, and saturated and *trans* fats), added sugars, and calories.

Both the USDA Food Guide and the DASH Eating Plan are constructed across a range of calorie levels to meet the nutrient needs of various age and gender groups.

KEY RECOMMENDATIONS

- Consume a variety of nutrient-dense foods and beverages within and among the basic food groups while choosing foods that limit the intake of saturated and *trans* fats, cholesterol, added sugars, salt, and alcohol.
- Meet recommended intakes within energy needs by adopting a balanced eating pattern, such as the USDA Food Guide or the DASH Eating Plan.

Key Recommendations for Specific Population Groups

- *People over age 50.* Consume vitamin B_{12} in its crystalline form (i.e., fortified foods or supplements).
- *Women of childbearing age who may become pregnant.* Eat foods high in heme-iron and/or consume iron-rich plant foods or iron-fortified foods with an enhancer of iron absorption, such as vitamin C-rich foods.
- *Women of childbearing age who may become pregnant and those in the first trimester of pregnancy.* Consume adequate synthetic folic acid daily (from fortified foods or supplements) in addition to food forms of folate from a varied diet.
- *Older adults, people with dark skin, and people exposed to insufficient ultraviolet band radiation (i.e., sunlight).* Consume extra vitamin D from vitamin D-fortified foods and/or supplements.

Table 1 (pages 265 to 266) provides food intake recommendations, and table 2 (page 267) provides nutrient profiles for both the DASH Eating Plan and the USDA Food Guide at the 2,000-calorie level. These tables illustrate the many similarities between the two eating patterns. Additional calorie levels are shown in appendixes A-1 and A-2 for the USDA Food Guide and the DASH Eating Plan. The exact amounts of foods in these plans do not need to be achieved every day, but on average, over time. Table 3 (page 268) can aid in identification of an individual's caloric requirement based on gender, age, and physical activity level.

Variety Among and Within Food Groups

Each basic food group[5] is the major contributor of at least one nutrient while making substantial contributions of many other nutrients. Because each food group provides a wide array of nutrients in substantial amounts, it is important to include all food groups in the daily diet.

---

[5] The food groups in the USDA Food Guide are grains; vegetables; fruits; milk, yogurt, and cheese; and meat, poultry, fish, dry beans, eggs, and nuts. Food groups in the DASH Eating Plan are grains and grain products; vegetables; fruits; low-fat or fat-free dairy; meat, poultry, and fish; and nuts, seeds, and dry beans.

Both illustrative eating patterns include a variety of nutrient-dense foods within the major food groups. Selecting a variety of foods within the grain, vegetable, fruit, and meat groups may help to ensure that an adequate amount of nutrients and other potentially beneficial substances are consumed. For example, fish contains varying amounts of fatty acids that may be beneficial in reducing cardiovascular disease risk (see Fats, pages 289 to 297).

Nutrient-Dense Foods

Nutrient-dense foods are those foods that provide substantial amounts of vitamins and minerals (micronutrients) and relatively few calories. Foods that are low in nutrient density are foods that supply calories but relatively small amounts of micronutrients, sometimes none at all. The greater the consumption of foods or beverages that are low in nutrient density, the more difficult it is to consume enough nutrients without gaining weight, especially for sedentary individuals. The consumption of added sugars, saturated and *trans* fats, and alcohol provides calories while providing little, if any, of the essential nutrients. (See Carbohydrates, pages 299 to 304 for additional information on added sugars, Fats, pages 289 to 297 for information on fats, and Alcoholic Beverages, pages 309 to 312 for information on alcohol.)

…meeting nutrient recommendations must go hand in hand with keeping calories under control.

Selecting low-fat forms of foods in each group and forms free of added sugars—in other words nutrient-dense versions of foods—provides individuals a way to meet their nutrient needs while avoiding the overconsumption of calories and of food components such as saturated fats. However, Americans generally do not eat nutrient-dense forms of foods. Most people will exceed calorie recommendations if they consistently choose higher fat foods within the food groups—even if they do not have dessert, sweetened beverages, or alcoholic beverages.

If only nutrient-dense foods are selected from each food group in the amounts proposed, a small amount of calories can be consumed as added fats or sugars, alcohol, or other foods—the *discretionary calorie allowance*. Appendixes A-2 and A-3 show the maximum discretionary calorie allowance that can be accommodated at each calorie level in the USDA Food Guide. Eating in accordance with the USDA Food Guide or the DASH Eating Plan will also keep intakes of saturated fat, total fat, and cholesterol within the limits recommended in Fats, pages 289 to 297.

Nutrients of Concern

The actual prevalence of inadequacy for a nutrient can be determined only if an Estimated Average Requirement (EAR) has been established and the distribution of usual dietary intake can be obtained. If such data are not available for a nutrient but there is evidence for a public health problem associated with low intakes, a nutrient might still be considered to be of concern.

Based on these considerations, dietary intakes of the following nutrients may be low enough to be of concern for:

- Adults: calcium, potassium, fiber, magnesium, and vitamins A (as carotenoids), C, and E,
- Children and adolescents: calcium, potassium, fiber, magnesium, and vitamin E,
- Specific population groups: vitamin B_{12}, iron, folic acid, and vitamins E and D.

Efforts may be warranted to promote increased dietary intakes of potassium, fiber, and possibly vitamin E, regardless of age; increased intakes of calcium and possibly vitamins A (as carotenoids) and C and magnesium by adults; efforts are warranted to increase intakes of calcium and possibly magnesium by children age 9 years or older. Efforts may be especially warranted to improve the dietary intakes of adolescent females in general. Food sources of these nutrients are shown in appendix B.

Low intakes of fiber tend to reflect low intakes of whole grains, fruits, and vegetables. Low intakes of calcium tend to reflect low intakes of milk and milk products. Low intakes of vitamins A (as carotenoids) and C and magnesium tend to reflect low intakes of fruits and vegetables. Selecting fruits, vegetables, whole grains, and low-fat and fat-free milk and milk products in the amounts suggested by the USDA Food Guide and the DASH Eating Plan will provide adequate amounts of these nutrients.

Most Americans of all ages also need to increase their potassium intake. To meet the recommended potassium intake levels, potassium-rich foods from the fruit, vegetable, and dairy groups must be selected in both the USDA Food Guide and the DASH Eating Plan. Foods that can help increase potassium intake are listed in table 5 (Food Groups to Encourage, page 286) and appendix B-1.

Most Americans may need to increase their consumption of foods rich in vitamin E (α-tocopherol) while decreasing their intake of foods high in energy but low in nutrients. The vitamin E content in both the USDA Food Guide and the DASH Eating Plan is greater than current consumption, and specific vitamin E-rich foods need to be included in the eating patterns to meet the recommended intake of vitamin E. Foods that can help increase vitamin E intake are listed in appendix B-2, along with their calorie content. Breakfast cereal that is fortified with vitamin E is an option for individuals seeking to increase their vitamin E intake while consuming a low-fat diet.

In addition, most Americans need to decrease sodium intake. The DASH Eating Plan provides guidance on how to keep sodium intakes within recommendations. When using the USDA Food Guide, selecting foods that are lower in sodium than others is especially necessary to meet the recommended intake level at calorie levels of 2,600/day and above. Food choices that are lower in sodium are identified in Sodium and Potassium, pages 305 to 308.

Considerations for Specific Population Groups

People Over 50 and Vitamin B_{12}

Although a substantial proportion of individuals over age 50 have reduced ability to absorb naturally occurring vitamin B_{12}, they are able to absorb the crystalline form. Thus, all individuals over the age of 50 should be encouraged to meet their Recommended Dietary Allowance (RDA) (2.4 µg/day) for vitamin B_{12} by eating foods fortified with vitamin B_{12} such as fortified cereals, or by taking the crystalline form of vitamin B_{12} supplements.

Women and Iron

Based on blood values, substantial numbers of adolescent females and women of childbearing age are iron deficient. Thus, these groups should eat foods high in heme-iron (e.g., meats) and/or consume iron-rich plant foods (e.g., spinach) or iron-fortified foods with an enhancer of iron absorption, such as foods rich in vitamin C (e.g., orange juice). Appendix B-3 lists foods that can help increase iron intake and gives their iron and calorie content.

Women and Folic Acid

Since folic acid reduces the risk of the neural tube defects, spina bifida, and anencephaly, a daily intake of 400 µg/day of synthetic folic acid (from fortified foods or supplements in addition to food forms of folate from a varied diet) is recommended for women of childbearing age who may become pregnant. Pregnant women should consume 600 µg/day of synthetic folic acid (from fortified foods or supplements) in addition to food forms of folate from a varied diet. It is not known whether the same level of protection could be achieved by using food that is naturally rich in folate.

Special Groups and Vitamin D

Adequate vitamin D status, which depends on dietary intake and cutaneous synthesis, is important for optimal calcium absorption, and it can reduce the risk for bone loss. Two functionally relevant measures indicate that optimal serum 25-hydroxyvitamin D may be as high as 80 nmol/L. The elderly and individuals with dark skin (because the ability to synthesize vitamin D from exposure to sunlight varies with degree of skin pigmentation) are at a greater risk of low serum 25-hydroxyvitamin D concentrations. Also at risk are those exposed to insufficient ultraviolet radiation (i.e., sunlight) for the cutaneous production of vitamin D (e.g., housebound individuals). For individuals within the high-risk groups, substantially higher daily intakes of vitamin D (i.e., 25 μg or 1,000 International Units (IU) of vitamin D per day) have been recommended to reach and maintain serum 25-hydroxyvitamin D values at 80 nmol/L. Three cups of vitamin D-fortified milk (7.5 μg or 300 IU), 1 cup of vitamin D-fortified orange juice (2.5 μg or 100 IU), and 15 μg (600 IU) of supplemental vitamin D would provide 25 μg (1,000 IU) of vitamin D daily.

Fluid

The combination of thirst and normal drinking behavior, especially the consumption of fluids with meals, is usually sufficient to maintain normal hydration. Healthy individuals who have routine access to fluids and who are not exposed to heat stress consume adequate water to meet their needs. Purposeful drinking is warranted for individuals who are exposed to heat stress or perform sustained vigorous activity (see Physical Activity, pages 277 to 280).

Flexibility of Food Patterns for Varied Food Preferences

The USDA Food Guide and the DASH Eating Plan are flexible to permit food choices based on individual and cultural food preferences, cost, and availability. Both can also accommodate varied types of cuisines and special needs due to common food allergies. Two adaptations of the USDA Food Guide and the DASH Eating Plan are:

Vegetarian Choices

Vegetarians of all types can achieve recommended nutrient intakes through careful selection of foods. These individuals should give special attention to their intakes of protein, iron, and vitamin B_{12}, as well as calcium and vitamin D if avoiding milk products. In addition, vegetarians could select only nuts, seeds, and legumes from the meat and beans group, or they could include eggs if so desired. At the 2,000-calorie level, they could choose about 1.5 ounces of nuts and $2/3$ cup legumes instead of 5.5 ounces of meat, poultry, and/or fish. One egg, $1/2$ ounce of nuts, or $1/4$ cup of legumes is considered equivalent to 1 ounce of meat, poultry, or fish in the USDA Food Guide.

Substitutions for Milk and Milk Products

Since milk and milk products provide more than 70 percent of the calcium consumed by Americans, guidance on other choices of dietary calcium is needed for those who do not consume the recommended amount of milk products. Milk product consumption has been associated with overall diet quality and adequacy of intake of many nutrients, including calcium, potassium, magnesium, zinc, iron, riboflavin, vitamin A, folate, and vitamin D. People may avoid milk products because of allergies, cultural practices, taste, or other reasons. Those who avoid all milk products need to choose rich sources of the nutrients provided by milk, including potassium, vitamin A, and magnesium in addition to calcium and vitamin D (see app. B). Some non-dairy sources of calcium are shown in appendix B-4. The bioavailability of the calcium in these foods varies.

Those who avoid milk because of its lactose content may obtain all the nutrients provided by the milk group by using lactose-reduced or low-lactose milk products, taking small servings of milk several times a day, taking the enzyme lactase before consuming milk products, or eating other calcium-rich foods. For additional information, see appendixes B-4 and B-5 and NIH Publication No. 03-2751.[6]

[6] NIH Publication No. 03-2751, U.S. Department of Health and Human Services, National Institutes of Health, National Institute of Diabetes and Digestive and Kidney Diseases, March 2003. http://digestive.niddk.nih.gov/ddiseases/pubs/lactoseintolerance/index.htm.

TABLE 1. Sample USDA Food Guide and the DASH Eating Plan at the 2,000-Calorie Level[a]

Amounts of various food groups that are recommended each day or each week in the USDA Food Guide and in the DASH Eating Plan (amounts are daily unless otherwise specified) at the 2,000-calorie level. Also identified are equivalent amounts for different food choices in each group. To follow either eating pattern, food choices over time should provide these amounts of food from each group on average.

Note: Table updated to reflect 2005 DASH Eating Plan.

Food Groups and Subgroups	USDA Food Guide Amount[b]	DASH Eating Plan Amount	Equivalent Amounts
Fruit Group	2 cups (4 servings)	2 to 2.5 cups (4 to 5 servings)	1/2 cup equivalent is: • 1/2 cup fresh, frozen, or canned fruit • 1 med fruit • 1/4 cup dried fruit • 1/2 cup fruit juice
Vegetable Group • Dark green vegetables • Orange vegetables • Legumes (dry beans) • Starchy vegetables • Other vegetables	2.5 cups (5 servings) 3 cups/week 2 cups/week 3 cups/week 3 cups/week 6.5 cups/week	2 to 2.5 cups (4 to 5 servings)	1/2 cup equivalent is: • 1/2 cup of cut-up raw or cooked vegetable • 1 cup raw leafy vegetable • 1/2 cup vegetable juice
Grain Group • Whole grains • Other grains	6 ounce-equivalents 3 ounce-equivalents 3 ounce-equivalents	6 to 8 ounce-equivalents (6 to 8 servings[c])	1 ounce-equivalent is: • 1 slice bread • 1 cup dry cereal • 1/2 cup cooked rice, pasta, cereal • DASH: 1 oz dry cereal (1/2–1 1/4 cup depending on cereal type—check label)
Meat and Beans Group	5.5 ounce-equivalents	6 ounces or less meats, poultry, fish	1 ounce-equivalent is: • 1 ounce of cooked lean meats, poultry, fish • 1 egg[e]
		4 to 5 servings per week nuts, seeds, and legumes[d]	• USDA: 1/4 cup cooked dry beans or tofu, 1 Tbsp peanut butter, 1/2 oz nuts or seeds • DASH: 1 1/2 oz nuts, 2 Tbsp peanut butter, 1/2 oz seeds, 1/2 cup cooked dry beans
Milk Group	3 cups	2 to 3 cups	1 cup equivalent is: • 1 cup low-fat/fat-free milk, yogurt • 1 1/2 oz of low-fat, fat-free, or reduced fat natural cheese • 2 oz of low-fat or fat-free processed cheese

Table 1 continues on page 266

TABLE 1: Continued

Food Groups and Subgroups	USDA Food Guide Amount[b]	DASH Eating Plan Amount	Equivalent Amounts
Oils	27 grams (6 tsp)	8 to 12 grams (2 to 3 tsp)	DASH: 1 tsp equivalent is: • 1 tsp soft margarine • 1 Tbsp low-fat mayo • 2 Tbsp light salad dressing • 1 tsp vegetable oil

Discretionary Calorie Allowance
• Example of distribution:
    Solid fat[f]
    Added sugars
	267 calories
	
	18 grams
	8 tsp
		
		~2 tsp (5 Tbsp per week)
			DASH: 1 Tbsp added sugar equivalent is:
			• 1 Tbsp jelly or jam
			• ½ cup sorbet and ices
			• 1 cup lemonade

[a] All servings are per day unless otherwise noted. USDA vegetable subgroup amounts and amounts of DASH nuts, seeds, and dry beans are per week.

[b] The 2,000-calorie USDA Food Guide is appropriate for many sedentary males 51 to 70 years of age, sedentary females 19 to 30 years of age, and for some other gender/age groups who are more physically active. See table 3 for information about gender/age/activity levels and appropriate calorie intakes. See appendixes A-2 and A-3 for more information on the food groups, amounts, and food intake patterns at other calorie levels.

[c] Whole grains are recommended for most grain servings to meet fiber recommendations.

[d] In the DASH Eating Plan, nuts, seeds, and legumes are a separate food group from meats, poultry, and fish.

[e] Since eggs are high in cholesterol, limit egg yolk intake to no more than 4 per week; 2 egg whites have the same protein content as 1 oz of meat.

[f] The oils listed in this table are not considered to be part of discretionary calories because they are a major source of vitamin E and polyunsaturated fatty acids, including the essential fatty acids, in the food pattern. In contrast, solid fats (i.e., saturated and *trans* fats) are listed separately as a source of discretionary calories.

TABLE 2. Comparison of Selected Nutrients in the DASH Eating Plan,[a] the USDA Food Guide,[b] and Nutrient Intakes Recommended Per Day by the Institute of Medicine (IOM)[c]

Estimated nutrient levels in the DASH Eating Plan and the USDA Food Guide at the 2,000-calorie level, as well as the nutrient intake levels recommended by the Institute of Medicine for females 19–30 years of age.

Note: Table updated to reflect 2005 DASH Eating Plan.

Nutrient	DASH Eating Plan (2,000 kcals)	USDA Food Guide (2,000 kcals)	IOM Recommendations for Females 19 to 30
Protein, g	105	91	RDA: 46
Protein, % kcal	20	18	AMDR: 10–35
Carbohydrate, g	281	271	RDA: 130
Carbohydrate, % kcal	54	55	AMDR: 45–65
Total fat, g	60	65	–
Total fat, % kcal	26	29	AMDR: 20–35
Saturated fat, g	12	17	–
Saturated fat, % kcal	6	7.8	ALAP[d]
Monounsaturated fat, g	25	24	–
Monounsaturated fat, % kcal	12	11	–
Polyunsaturated fat, g	16	20	–
Polyunsaturated fat, % kcal	7	9.0	–
Linoleic acid, g	14	18	AI: 12
Alpha-linolenic acid, g	2.2	1.7	AI: 1.1
Cholesterol, mg	136	230	ALAP[d]
Total dietary fiber, g	34	31	AI: 28[e]
Potassium, mg	4,721	4,044	AI: 4,700
Sodium, mg	2,096[f]	1,779	AI: 1,500, UL: <2,300
Calcium, mg	1,406	1,316	AI: 1,000
Magnesium, mg	554	380	RDA: 310
Copper, mg	1.9	1.5	RDA: 0.9
Iron, mg	22	18	RDA: 18
Phosphorus, mg	1,955	1,740	RDA: 700
Zinc, mg	14	14	RDA: 8
Thiamin, mg	1.7	2.0	RDA: 1.1
Riboflavin, mg	2.7	2.8	RDA: 1.1
Niacin equivalents, mg	50	22	RDA: 14
Vitamin B_6, mg	2.9	2.4	RDA: 1.3
Vitamin B_{12}, µg	5.6	8.3	RDA: 2.4
Vitamin C, mg	162	155	RDA: 75
Vitamin E (AT)[g]	19	9.5	RDA: 15.0
Vitamin A, µg (RAE)[h]	925	1,052	RDA: 700

[a] DASH nutrient values are based on a 1-week menu of the DASH Eating Plan. Visit www.nhlbi.nih.gov.

[b] USDA nutrient values are based on population-weighted averages of typical food choices within each food group or subgroup.

[c] Recommended intakes for adult females 19–30; RDA = Recommended Dietary Allowance; AI = Adequate Intake; AMDR = Acceptable Macronutrient Distribution Range; UL = Upper Limit.

[d] As Low As Possible while consuming a nutritionally adequate diet.

[e] Amount listed is based on 14 g dietary fiber/1,000 kcal.

[f] The DASH Eating Plan also can be used to follow at 1,500 mg sodium per day.

[g] AT = mg d-α-tocopherol

[h] RAE = Retinol Activity Equivalents

TABLE 3. Estimated Calorie Requirements (in Kilocalories) for Each Gender and Age Group at Three Levels of Physical Activity[a]

Estimated amounts of calories needed to maintain energy balance for various gender and age groups at three different levels of physical activity. The estimates are rounded to the nearest 200 calories and were determined using the Institute of Medicine equation.

Gender	Age (years)	Activity Level[b,c,d]		
		Sedentary[b]	Moderately Active[c]	Active[d]
Child	2–3	1,000	1,000–1,400[e]	1,000–1,400[e]
Female	4–8	1,200	1,400–1,600	1,400–1,800
	9–13	1,600	1,600–2,000	1,800–2,200
	14–18	1,800	2,000	2,400
	19–30	2,000	2,000–2,200	2,400
	31–50	1,800	2,000	2,200
	51+	1,600	1,800	2,000–2,200
Male	4–8	1,400	1,400–1,600	1,600–2,000
	9–13	1,800	1,800–2,200	2,000–2,600
	14–18	2,200	2,400–2,800	2,800–3,200
	19–30	2,400	2,600–2,800	3,000
	31–50	2,200	2,400–2,600	2,800–3,000
	51+	2,000	2,200–2,400	2,400–2,800

[a] These levels are based on Estimated Energy Requirements (EER) from the Institute of Medicine Dietary Reference Intakes macronutrients report, 2002, calculated by gender, age, and activity level for reference-sized individuals. "Reference size," as determined by IOM, is based on median height and weight for ages up to age 18 years of age and median height and weight for that height to give a BMI of 21.5 for adult females and 22.5 for adult males.

[b] Sedentary means a lifestyle that includes only the light physical activity associated with typical day-to-day life.

[c] Moderately active means a lifestyle that includes physical activity equivalent to walking about 1.5 to 3 miles per day at 3 to 4 miles per hour, in addition to the light physical activity associated with typical day-to-day life.

[d] Active means a lifestyle that includes physical activity equivalent to walking more than 3 miles per day at 3 to 4 miles per hour, in addition to the light physical activity associated with typical day-to-day life.

[e] The calorie ranges shown are to accommodate needs of different ages within the group. For children and adolescents, more calories are needed at older ages. For adults, fewer calories are needed at older ages.

Weight Management

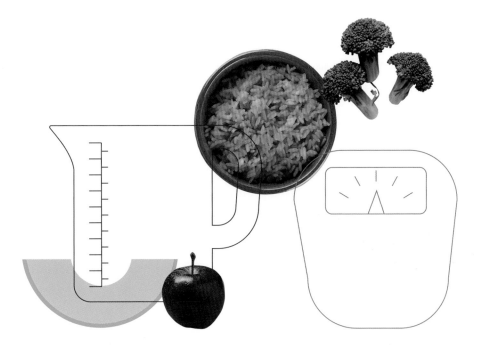

OVERVIEW

The prevalence of obesity in the United States has doubled in the past two decades. Nearly one-third of adults are obese, that is, they have a body mass index (BMI) of 30 or greater. One of the fastest growing segments of the population is that with a BMI≥30 with accompanying comorbidities. Over the last two decades, the prevalence of overweight among children and adolescents has increased substantially; it is estimated that as many as 16 percent of children and adolescents are overweight, representing a doubling of the rate among children and tripling of the rate among adolescents. A high prevalence of overweight and obesity is of great public health concern because excess body fat leads to a higher risk for premature death, type 2 diabetes, hypertension, dyslipidemia, cardiovascular disease, stroke, gall bladder disease, respiratory dysfunction, gout, osteoarthritis, and certain kinds of cancers.

Ideally, the goal for adults is to achieve and maintain a body weight that optimizes their health. However, for obese adults, even modest weight loss (e.g., 10 pounds) has health benefits, and the prevention of further weight gain is very important. For overweight children and adolescents, the goal is to slow the rate of weight gain while achieving normal growth and development. Maintaining a healthy weight throughout childhood may reduce the risk of becoming an overweight or obese adult. Eating fewer calories while increasing physical activity are the keys to controlling body weight.

While overweight and obesity are currently significant public health issues, not all Americans need to lose weight. People at a healthy weight should strive to maintain their weight, and underweight individuals may need to increase their weight.

DISCUSSION

Overweight and obesity in the United States among adults and children has increased significantly over the last two decades. Those following typical American eating and activity patterns are likely to be consuming diets in excess of their energy requirements. However, caloric intake is only one side of the energy balance equation. Caloric expenditure needs to be in balance with caloric intake to maintain body weight and must exceed caloric intake to achieve weight loss (see table 3, page 268, and table 4, page 273). To reverse the trend toward obesity, most Americans need to eat fewer calories, be more active, and make wiser food choices.

Prevention of weight gain is critical because while the behaviors required are the same, the extent of the behaviors required to lose weight makes weight loss more challenging than prevention of weight gain. Since many adults gain weight slowly over time, even small decreases in calorie intake can help avoid weight gain, especially if accompanied by increased physical activity. For example, for most adults a reduction of 50 to 100 calories per day may prevent gradual weight gain, whereas a reduction of 500 calories or more per day is a common initial goal in weight-loss programs. Similarly, up to 60 minutes of moderate- to vigorous-intensity physical activity per day may be needed to prevent weight gain, but as much as 60 to 90 minutes of moderate-intensity physical activity per day is recommended to sustain weight loss for previously overweight people. It is advisable for men over age 40, women over age 50, and those with a history of chronic diseases such as heart disease or diabetes to consult with a healthcare provider before starting a vigorous exercise program. However, many people can safely increase their physical activity without consulting a healthcare provider.[7]

[7] For more information on recommendations to consult a healthcare provider, see Physical Activity and Public Health—A Recommendation from the Centers for Disease Control and Prevention and the American College of Sports Medicine, *JAMA* 273:402-407, 1995. http://wonder.cdc.gov/wonder/prevguid/p0000391/P0000391.asp.

KEY RECOMMENDATIONS

- To maintain body weight in a healthy range, balance calories from foods and beverages with calories expended.
- To prevent gradual weight gain over time, make small decreases in food and beverage calories and increase physical activity.

Key Recommendations for Specific Population Groups

- *Those who need to lose weight.* Aim for a slow, steady weight loss by decreasing calorie intake while maintaining an adequate nutrient intake and increasing physical activity.
- *Overweight children.* Reduce the rate of body weight gain while allowing growth and development. Consult a healthcare provider before placing a child on a weight-reduction diet.
- *Pregnant women.* Ensure appropriate weight gain as specified by a healthcare provider.
- *Breastfeeding women.* Moderate weight reduction is safe and does not compromise weight gain of the nursing infant.
- *Overweight adults and overweight children with chronic diseases and/or on medication.* Consult a healthcare provider about weight loss strategies prior to starting a weight-reduction program to ensure appropriate management of other health conditions.

Monitoring body fat regularly can be a useful strategy for assessing the need to adjust caloric intake and energy expenditure. Two surrogate measures used to approximate body fat are BMI (adults and children) and waist circumference (adults).[8] BMI is defined as weight in kilograms divided by height, in meters, squared. For adults, weight status is based on the absolute BMI level (fig. 2, page 274). For children and adolescents, weight status is determined by the comparison of the individual's BMI with age- and gender-specific percentile values (see fig. 3, page 275, for a sample boys' growth curve). Additional growth curves can be found at http://www.cdc.gov/growthcharts. BMI is more accurate at approximating body fat than is measuring body weight alone. However, BMI has some limitations. BMI overestimates body fat in people who are very muscular and underestimates body fat in people who have lost muscle mass. The relationship between BMI and body fat varies somewhat with age, gender, and ethnicity. In addition, for adults, BMI is a better predictor of a population's disease risk than an individual's risk of chronic disease.[8] For children gaining

---

[8] NIH Publication Number 00-4084, The Practical Guide: Identification, Evaluation and Treatment of Overweight and Obesity in Adults, U.S. Department of Health and Human Services, National Institutes of Health, National Heart, Lung, and Blood Institute, October 2000. http://www.nhlbi.nih.gov/guidelines/obesity/prctgd_c.pdf.

excess weight, small decreases in energy intake reduce the rate at which they gain weight (body fat), thus improving their BMI percentile over time. As another surrogate measure, waist circumference can approximate abdominal fat but should be measured very carefully. Fat located in the abdominal region is associated with a greater health risk than peripheral fat.[8]

Some proposed calorie-lowering strategies include eating foods that are low in calories for a given measure of food (e.g., many kinds of vegetables and fruits and some soups). However, when making changes to improve nutrient intake, one needs to make substitutions to avoid excessive calorie intake. The healthiest way to reduce calorie intake is to reduce one's intake of added sugars, fats, and alcohol, which all provide calories but few or no essential nutrients (for more information, see "Fats," page 289; "Carbohydrates," page 299; and "Sodium and Potassium," page 305).

Eating fewer calories while increasing physical activity are the keys to controlling body weight.

Special attention should be given to portion sizes, which have increased significantly over the past two decades (http://hin.nhlbi.nih.gov/portion/index.htm). Though there are no empirical studies to show a causal relationship between increased portion sizes and obesity, there are studies showing that controlling portion sizes helps limit calorie intake, particularly when eating calorie-dense foods (foods that are high in calories for a given measure of food). Therefore, it is essential that the public understand how portion sizes compare to a recommended amount of food (i.e., serving) from each food group at a specific caloric level. The understanding of serving size and portion size is important in following either the DASH Eating Plan or the USDA Food Guide (see app. A). When using packaged foods with nutrient labels, people should pay attention to the units for serving sizes and how they compare to the serving sizes in the USDA Food Guide and the DASH Eating Plan.

Lifestyle change in diet and physical activity is the best first choice for weight loss. A reduction in 500 calories or more per day is commonly needed. When it comes to body weight control, it is calories that count—not the proportions of fat,

---

[8] NIH Publication Number 00-4084, The Practical Guide: Identification, Evaluation and Treatment of Overweight and Obesity in Adults, U.S. Department of Health and Human Services, National Institutes of Health, National Heart, Lung, and Blood Institute, October 2000. http://www.nhlbi.nih.gov/guidelines/obesity/prctgd_c.pdf.

carbohydrates, and protein in the diet. However, when individuals are losing weight, they should follow a diet that is within the Acceptable Macronutrient Distribution Ranges (AMDR) for fat, carbohydrates, and protein, which are 20 to 35 percent of total calories, 45 to 65 percent of total calories, and 10 to 35 percent of total calories, respectively. Diets that provide very low or very high amounts of protein, carbohydrates, or fat are likely to provide low amounts of some nutrients and are not advisable for long term use. Although these kinds of weight-loss diets have been shown to result in weight reduction, the maintenance of a reduced weight ultimately will depend on a change in lifestyle. Successful and sustainable weight loss and weight maintenance strategies require attention to both sides of the energy balance equation (i.e., caloric intake and energy expenditure).

TABLE 4. Calories/Hour Expended in Common Physical Activities

Some examples of physical activities commonly engaged in and the average amount of calories a 154-pound individual will expend by engaging in each activity for 1 hour. The expenditure value encompasses both resting metabolic rate calories and activity expenditure. Some of the activities can constitute either moderate- or vigorous-intensity physical activity depending on the rate at which they are carried out (for walking and bicycling).

Moderate Physical Activity	Approximate Calories/Hr for a 154 lb Person[a]
Hiking	370
Light gardening/yard work	330
Dancing	330
Golf (walking and carrying clubs)	330
Bicycling (<10 mph)	290
Walking (3.5 mph)	280
Weight lifting (general light workout)	220
Stretching	180
Vigorous Physical Activity	**Approximate Calories/Hr for a 154 lb Person[a]**
Running/jogging (5 mph)	590
Bicycling (>10 mph)	590
Swimming (slow freestyle laps)	510
Aerobics	480
Walking (4.5 mph)	460
Heavy yard work (chopping wood)	440
Weight lifting (vigorous effort)	440
Basketball (vigorous)	440

[a] Calories burned per hour will be higher for persons who weigh more than 154 lbs (70 kg) and lower for persons who weigh less.
Source: Adapted from the 2005 DGAC Report.

FIGURE 2. Adult BMI Chart

Locate the height of interest in the left-most column and read across the row for that height to the weight of interest. Follow the column of the weight up to the top row that lists the BMI. BMI of 18.5–24.9 is the healthy weight range, BMI of 25–29.9 is the overweight range, and BMI of 30 and above is in the obese range.

BMI	19	20	21	22	23	24	25	26	27	28	29	30	31	32	33	34	35
Height							Weight in Pounds										
4'10"	91	96	100	105	110	115	119	124	129	134	138	143	148	153	158	162	167
4'11"	94	99	104	109	114	119	124	128	133	138	143	148	153	158	163	168	173
5'	97	102	107	112	118	123	128	133	138	143	148	153	158	163	158	174	179
5'1"	100	106	111	116	122	127	132	137	143	148	153	158	164	169	174	180	185
5'2"	104	109	115	120	126	131	136	142	147	153	158	164	169	175	180	186	191
5'3"	107	113	118	124	130	135	141	146	152	158	163	169	175	180	186	191	197
5'4"	110	116	122	128	134	140	145	151	157	163	169	174	180	186	192	197	204
5'5"	114	120	126	132	138	144	150	156	162	168	174	180	186	192	198	204	210
5'6"	118	124	130	136	142	148	155	161	167	173	179	186	192	198	204	210	216
5'7"	121	127	134	140	146	153	159	166	172	178	185	191	198	204	211	217	223
5'8"	125	131	138	144	151	158	164	171	177	184	190	197	203	210	216	223	230
5'9"	128	135	142	149	155	162	169	176	182	189	196	203	209	216	223	230	236
5'10"	132	139	146	153	160	167	174	181	188	195	202	209	216	222	229	236	243
5'11"	136	143	150	157	165	172	179	186	193	200	208	215	222	229	236	243	250
6'	140	147	154	162	169	177	184	191	199	206	213	221	228	235	242	250	258
6'1"	144	151	159	166	174	182	189	197	204	212	219	227	235	242	250	257	265
6'2'	148	155	163	171	179	186	194	202	210	218	225	233	241	249	256	264	272
6'3'	152	160	168	176	184	192	200	208	216	224	232	240	248	256	264	272	279
	Healthy Weight						Overweight					Obese					

Source: Evidence Report of Clinical Guidelines on the Identification, Evaluation, and Treatment of Overweight and Obesity in Adults, 1998. NIH/National Heart, Lung, and Blood Institute (NHLBI).

FIGURE 3. Example of Boys' BMI Growth Curve (2 to 20 years): Boys' Body Mass Index-For-Age Percentiles

Calculate the BMI for an individual child using the following:

BMI = Weight (kg)/(Height [cm])² x 10,000 or BMI = Weight (lb)/(Height [in])² x 703

Find the age of the child on the bottom, x-axis, and read up the chart from that age to the calculated BMI on the left and right, y-axis. The curve that is closest to the spot where the age and BMI of the child meet on the graph indicate the BMI percentile for this child relative to the population.

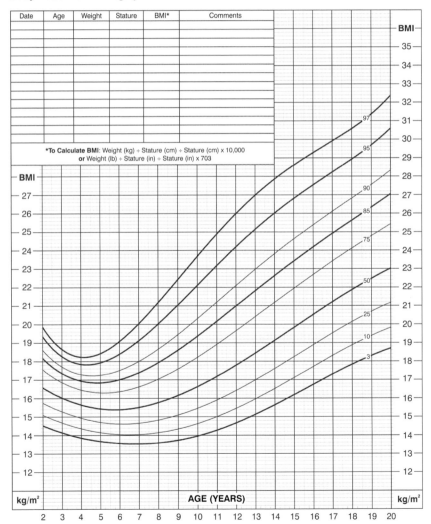

Published May 30, 2000 (modified 10/16/00).

Source: Developed by the National Center for Health Statistics in collaboration with the National Center for Chronic Disease Prevention and Health Promotion. http://www.cdc.gov/growthcharts (2000). Other growth charts are available at this source.

Physical Activity

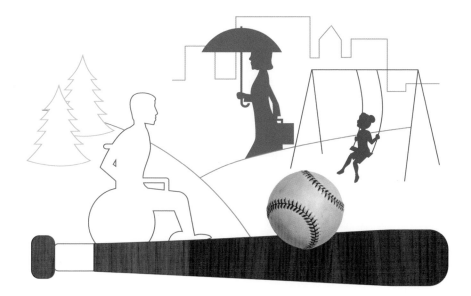

OVERVIEW

Americans tend to be relatively inactive. In 2002, 25 percent of adult Americans did not participate in any leisure time physical activities in the past month,[9] and in 2003, 38 percent of students in grades 9 to 12 viewed television 3 or more hours per day.[10] Regular physical activity and physical fitness make important contributions to one's health, sense of well-being, and maintenance of a healthy body weight. Physical activity is defined as any bodily movement produced by skeletal muscles resulting in energy expenditure (http://www.cdc.gov/nccdphp/dnpa/physical/terms/index.htm). In contrast, physical fitness is a multi-component trait related to the ability to perform physical activity. Maintenance of good physical fitness enables one to meet the physical demands of work and leisure comfortably. People with higher levels of physical

9 Behavioral Risk Factor Surveillance System, Surveillance for Certain Health Behaviors Among Selected Local Areas—United States, Behavioral Risk Factor Surveillance System, 2002, *Morbidity and Mortality Weekly Report (MMWR)*, 53, No SS-05. http://www.cdc.gov/brfss/.

10 Youth Risk Behavior Surveillance System, Youth Risk Behavior Surveillance—United States, 2003 *MMWR* 53(SS-2):1–29, 2004. http://www.cdc.gov/healthyyouth/yrbs/.

fitness are also at lower risk of developing chronic disease. Conversely, a sedentary lifestyle increases risk for overweight and obesity and many chronic diseases, including coronary artery disease, hypertension, type 2 diabetes, osteoporosis, and certain types of cancer. Overall, mortality rates from all causes of death are lower in physically active people than in sedentary people. Also, physical activity can aid in managing mild to moderate depression and anxiety.

DISCUSSION

Regular physical activity has been shown to reduce the risk of certain chronic diseases, including high blood pressure, stroke, coronary artery disease, type 2 diabetes, colon cancer and osteoporosis. Therefore, to reduce the risk of chronic disease, it is recommended that adults engage in at least 30 minutes of moderate-intensity physical activity on most, preferably all, days of the week. For most people, greater health benefits can be obtained by engaging in physical activity of more vigorous intensity or of longer duration. In addition, physical activity appears to promote psychological well-being and reduce feelings of mild to moderate depression and anxiety.

Regular physical activity is also a key factor in achieving and maintaining a healthy body weight for adults and children. To prevent the gradual accumulation of excess weight in adulthood, up to 30 additional minutes per day may be required over the 30 minutes for reduction of chronic disease risk and other health benefits. That is, approximately 60 minutes of moderate- to vigorous-intensity physical activity on most days of the week may be needed to prevent unhealthy weight gain (see table 4, page 273, for some examples of moderate- and vigorous-intensity physical activities). While moderate-intensity physical activity can achieve the desired goal, vigorous-intensity physical activity generally provides more benefits than moderate-intensity physical activity. Control of caloric intake is also advisable. However, to sustain weight loss for previously overweight/obese people, about 60 to 90 minutes of moderate-intensity physical activity per day is recommended.

Most adults do not need to see their healthcare provider before starting a moderate-intensity physical activity program. However, men older than 40 years and women older than 50 years who plan a vigorous program or who have either chronic disease or risk factors for chronic disease should consult their physician to design a safe, effective program. It is also important during leisure time to limit sedentary behaviors, such as television watching and video viewing, and replace them with activities requiring more movement. Reducing these sedentary activities appears to be helpful in treating and preventing overweight among children and adolescents.

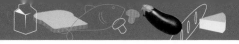
KEY RECOMMENDATIONS

- Engage in regular physical activity and reduce sedentary activities to promote health, psychological well-being, and a healthy body weight.
  - To reduce the risk of chronic disease in adulthood: Engage in at least 30 minutes of moderate-intensity physical activity, above usual activity, at work or home on most days of the week.
  - For most people, greater health benefits can be obtained by engaging in physical activity of more vigorous intensity or longer duration.
  - To help manage body weight and prevent gradual, unhealthy body weight gain in adulthood: Engage in approximately 60 minutes of moderate- to vigorous-intensity activity on most days of the week while not exceeding caloric intake requirements.
  - To sustain weight loss in adulthood: Participate in at least 60 to 90 minutes of daily moderate-intensity physical activity while not exceeding caloric intake requirements. Some people may need to consult with a healthcare provider before participating in this level of activity.
- Achieve physical fitness by including cardiovascular conditioning, stretching exercises for flexibility, and resistance exercises or calisthenics for muscle strength and endurance.

Key Recommendations for Specific Population Groups
- *Children and adolescents.* Engage in at least 60 minutes of physical activity on most, preferably all, days of the week.
- *Pregnant women.* In the absence of medical or obstetric complications, incorporate 30 minutes or more of moderate-intensity physical activity on most, if not all, days of the week. Avoid activities with a high risk of falling or abdominal trauma.
- *Breastfeeding women.* Be aware that neither acute nor regular exercise adversely affects the mother's ability to successfully breastfeed.
- *Older adults.* Participate in regular physical activity to reduce functional declines associated with aging and to achieve the other benefits of physical activity identified for all adults.

Different intensities and types of exercise confer different benefits. Vigorous physical activity (e.g., jogging or other aerobic exercise) provides greater benefits for physical fitness than does moderate physical activity and burns more calories per unit of time. Resistance exercise (such as weight training, using weight machines, and resistance band workouts) increases muscular strength and endurance and maintains or increases muscle mass. These benefits are seen in adolescents, adults, and older adults who perform resistance exercises on 2 or more days per week. Also, weight-bearing exercise has the potential to reduce the risk of osteoporosis by increasing peak bone mass during growth, maintaining peak bone mass during adulthood, and reducing the rate of bone loss during aging. In addition, regular exercise can help prevent falls, which is of particular importance for older adults.

The barrier often given for a failure to be physically active is lack of time. Setting aside 30 to 60 consecutive minutes each day for planned exercise is one way to obtain physical activity, but it is not the only way. Physical activity may include short bouts (e.g., 10-minute bouts) of moderate-intensity activity. The accumulated total is what is important—both for health and for burning calories. Physical activity can be accumulated through three to six 10-minute bouts over the course of a day.

Elevating the level of daily physical activity may also provide indirect nutritional benefits. A sedentary lifestyle limits the number of calories that can be consumed without gaining weight. The higher a person's physical activity level, the higher his or her energy requirement and the easier it is to plan a daily food intake pattern that meets recommended nutrient requirements.

Proper hydration is important when participating in physical activity. Two steps that help avoid dehydration during prolonged physical activity or when it is hot include: (1) consuming fluid regularly during the activity and (2) drinking several glasses of water or other fluid after the physical activity is completed (see Nutrient Adequacy, pages 257 to 268).

Regular physical activity and physical fitness make important contributions to one's health, sense of well-being, and maintenance of a healthy body weight.

Food Groups To Encourage

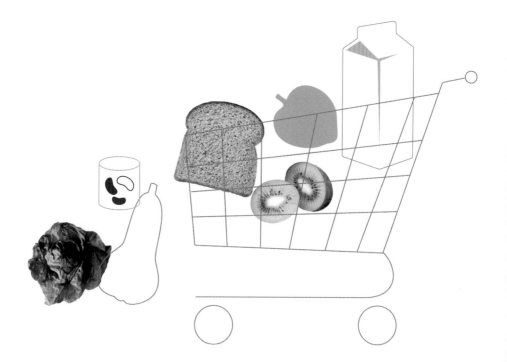

OVERVIEW

Increased intakes of fruits, vegetables, whole grains, and fat-free or low-fat milk and milk products are likely to have important health benefits for most Americans. While protein is an important macronutrient in the diet, most Americans are already currently consuming enough (AMDR = 10 to 35 percent of calories) and do not need to increase their intake. As such, protein consumption, while important for nutrient adequacy, is not a focus of this document. Although associations have been identified between specific food groups (e.g., fruits and vegetables) and reduced risk for chronic diseases, the effects are interrelated and the health benefits should be considered in the context of an overall healthy diet that does not exceed calorie needs (such as the USDA Food Guide or the DASH Eating Plan; see Nutrient Adequacy, pages 257 to 268). The strength of the evidence for the association between increased intake of fruits and vegetables and reduced risk of chronic diseases is variable and depends on the specific disease, but an array of evidence points to beneficial health effects.

Compared with the many people who consume a dietary pattern with only small amounts of fruits and vegetables, those who eat more generous amounts as part of a healthful diet are likely to have reduced risk of chronic diseases, including stroke and perhaps other cardiovascular diseases, type 2 diabetes, and cancers in certain sites (oral cavity and pharynx, larynx, lung, esophagus, stomach, and colon-rectum). Diets rich in foods containing fiber, such as fruits, vegetables, and whole grains, may reduce the risk of coronary heart disease. Diets rich in milk and milk products can reduce the risk of low bone mass throughout the life cycle. The consumption of milk products is especially important for children and adolescents who are building their peak bone mass and developing lifelong habits. Although each of these food groups may have a different relationship with disease outcomes, the adequate consumption of all food groups contributes to overall health.

DISCUSSION

Fruits, vegetables, whole grains, and milk products are all important to a healthful diet and can be good sources of the nutrients of concern (see Nutrient Adequacy, pages 257 to 268). When increasing intake of fruits, vegetables, whole grains, and fat-free or low-fat milk and milk products, it is important to decrease one's intake of less-nutrient-dense foods to control calorie intake. The 2,000-calorie level used in the discussion is a reference level only; it is not a recommended calorie intake because many Americans should be consuming fewer calories to maintain a healthy weight.

Fruits and Vegetables

Four and one-half cups (nine servings) of fruits and vegetables are recommended daily for the reference 2,000-calorie level, with higher or lower amounts depending on the caloric level. This results in a range of 2½ to 6½ cups (5 to 13 servings) of fruits and vegetables each day for the 1,200- to 3,200-calorie levels[11] (app. A-2). Fruits and vegetables provide a variety of micronutrients and fiber. Table 5 (page 286) provides a list of fruits and vegetables that are good sources of vitamins A (as carotenoids) and C, folate, and potassium. In the fruit group, consumption of whole fruits (fresh, frozen, canned, dried) rather than fruit juice for the majority of the total daily amount is suggested to ensure adequate fiber intake. Different vegetables are rich in different nutrients. In the vegetable group, weekly intake of specific amounts from each of five vegetable subgroups (dark green, orange, legumes [dry beans], starchy, and other vegetables)[12] is recommended for adequate nutrient intake.

[11] See appendix A-2 and table D1-16 from the 2005 DGAC Report (or USDA website) for information on children age 2 to 3 years.

[12] Includes all fresh, frozen, canned, cooked, or raw forms of vegetables. Examples of vegetables are dark green (broccoli, spinach, most greens); orange (carrots, sweetpotatoes, winter squash, pumpkin); legumes (dry beans, chickpeas, tofu); starchy (corn, white potatoes, green peas); other (tomatoes, cabbage, celery, cucumber, lettuce, onions, peppers, green beans, cauliflower, mushrooms, summer squash).

Each subgroup provides a somewhat different array of nutrients. In the USDA Food Guide at the reference 2,000-calorie level, the following weekly amounts are recommended:

Dark green vegetables	3 cups/week
Orange vegetables	2 cups/week
Legumes (dry beans)	3 cups/week
Starchy vegetables	3 cups/week
Other vegetables	6½ cups/week

Most current consumption patterns do not achieve the recommended intakes of many of these vegetables. The DASH Eating Plan and the USDA Food Guide suggest increasing intakes of dark green vegetables, orange vegetables, and legumes (dry beans) as part of the overall recommendation to have an adequate intake of fruits and vegetables (see Nutrient Adequacy, pages 257 to 268).

KEY RECOMMENDATIONS

- Consume a sufficient amount of fruits and vegetables while staying within energy needs. Two cups of fruit and 2½ cups of vegetables per day are recommended for a reference 2,000-calorie intake, with higher or lower amounts depending on the calorie level.
- Choose a variety of fruits and vegetables each day. In particular, select from all five vegetable subgroups (dark green, orange, legumes, starchy vegetables, and other vegetables) several times a week.
- Consume 3 or more ounce-equivalents of whole-grain products per day, with the rest of the recommended grains coming from enriched or whole-grain products. In general, at least half the grains should come from whole grains.
- Consume 3 cups per day of fat-free or low-fat milk or equivalent milk products.

Key Recommendations for Specific Population Groups

- *Children and adolescents*. Consume whole-grain products often; at least half the grains should be whole grains. Children 2 to 8 years should consume 2 cups per day of fat-free or low-fat milk or equivalent milk products. Children 9 years of age and older should consume 3 cups per day of fat-free or low-fat milk or equivalent milk products.

Whole Grains

In addition to fruits and vegetables, whole grains are an important source of fiber and other nutrients. Whole grains, as well as foods made from them, consist of the entire grain seed, usually called the kernel. The kernel is made of three components— the bran, the germ, and the endosperm. If the kernel has been cracked, crushed, or flaked, then it must retain nearly the same relative proportions of bran, germ, and endosperm as the original grain to be called whole grain. In the grain-refining process, most of the bran and some of the germ is removed, resulting in the loss of dietary fiber (also known as cereal fiber), vitamins, minerals, lignans, phytoestrogens, phenolic compounds, and phytic acid. Some manufacturers add bran to grain products to increase the dietary fiber content. Refined grains are the resulting product of the grain-refining processing. Most refined grains are enriched before being further processed into foods. Enriched refined grain products that conform to standards of identity are required by law to be fortified with folic acid, as well as thiamin, ribo-flavin, niacin, and iron. Food manufacturers may fortify whole-grain foods where regulations permit the addition of folic acid. Currently, a number of whole-grain, ready-to-eat breakfast cereals are fortified with folic acid. As illustrated by the comparison of whole-wheat and enriched white flours in table 6 (page 287), many nutrients occur at higher or similar levels in whole grains when compared to enriched grains, but whole grains have less folate unless they have been fortified with folic acid.

Increased intakes of fruits, vegetables, whole grains, and fat-free or low-fat milk and milk products are likely to have important health benefits for most Americans.

Consuming at least 3 or more ounce-equivalents of whole grains per day can reduce the risk of several chronic diseases and may help with weight maintenance. Thus, daily intake of at least 3 ounce-equivalents of whole grains per day is recommended by substituting whole grains for refined grains. However, because three servings may be difficult for younger children to achieve, it is recommended that they increase whole grains into their diets as they grow. At all calorie levels, all age groups should consume at least half the grains as whole grains to achieve the fiber recommendation. All grain servings can be whole-grain; however, it is advisable to include some folate-fortified products, such as folate-fortified whole-grain cereals, in these whole-grain choices.

Whole grains cannot be identified by the color of the food; label-reading skills are needed. Table 7 (page 288) identifies names of whole grains that are available in the United States. For information about the ingredients in whole-grain and enriched-grain products, read the ingredient list on the food label. For many whole-grain products, the words "whole" or "whole grain" will appear before the grain ingredient's name. The whole grain should be the first ingredient listed. Wheat flour, enriched flour, and degerminated cornmeal are not whole grains. The Food and Drug Administration requires foods that bear the whole-grain health claim to (1) contain 51 percent or more whole-grain ingredients by weight per reference amount and (2) be low in fat.

Milk and Milk Products

Another source of nutrients is milk and milk products. Milk product consumption has been associated with overall diet quality and adequacy of intake of many nutrients. The intake of milk products is especially important to bone health during childhood and adolescence. Studies specifically on milk and other milk products, such as yogurt and cheese, showed a positive relationship between the intake of milk and milk products and bone mineral content or bone mineral density in one or more skeletal sites (see table 1, page 265, for information on equivalent amounts of milk products).

Adults and children should not avoid milk and milk products because of concerns that these foods lead to weight gain. There are many fat-free and low-fat choices without added sugars that are available and consistent with an overall healthy dietary plan. If a person wants to consider milk alternatives because of lactose intolerance, the most reliable and easiest ways to derive the health benefits associated with milk and milk product consumption are to choose alternatives within the milk food group, such as yogurt or lactose-free milk, or to consume the enzyme lactase prior to the consumption of milk products. For individuals who choose to or must avoid all milk products (e.g., individuals with lactose intolerance, vegans), non-dairy calcium-containing alternatives may be selected to help meet calcium needs (app. B-4).

TABLE 5. Fruits, Vegetables, and Legumes (Dry Beans) That Contain Vitamin A (Carotenoids), Vitamin C, Folate, and Potassium

Many of the fruits, vegetables, and legumes (beans) are considered to be important sources of vitamin A (as carotenoids), vitamin C, and potassium in the adult population. Intakes of these nutrients, based on dietary intake data or evidence of public health problems, may be of concern. Also listed are sources of naturally occurring folate, a nutrient considered to be of concern for women of childbearing age and those in the first trimester of pregnancy. Folic acid-fortified grain products, not listed in this table, are also good sources.

Sources of vitamin A (carotenoids) (see app. B-6)
- Bright orange vegetables like carrots, sweetpotatoes, and pumpkin
- Tomatoes and tomato products, red sweet pepper
- Leafy greens such as spinach, collards, turnip greens, kale, beet and mustard greens, green leaf lettuce, and romaine
- Orange fruits like mango, cantaloupe, apricots, and red or pink grapefruit

Sources of vitamin C
- Citrus fruits and juices, kiwi fruit, strawberries, guava, papaya, and cantaloupe
- Broccoli, peppers, tomatoes, cabbage (especially Chinese cabbage), brussels sprouts, and potatoes
- Leafy greens such as romaine, turnip greens, and spinach

Sources of folate
- Cooked dry beans and peas
- Oranges and orange juice
- Deep green leaves like spinach and mustard greens

Sources of potassium (see app. B-1)
- Baked white or sweetpotatoes, cooked greens (such as spinach), winter (orange) squash
- Bananas, plantains, many dried fruits, oranges and orange juice, cantaloupe, and honeydew melons
- Cooked dry beans
- Soybeans (green and mature)
- Tomato products (sauce, paste, puree)
- Beet greens

TABLE 6. Comparison of 100 Grams of Whole-Grain Wheat Flour and Enriched, Bleached, White, All-Purpose Flour

Some of the nutrients of concern and the fortification nutrients in 100 percent whole-wheat flour and enriched, bleached, all-purpose white (wheat) flour. Dietary fiber, calcium, magnesium and potassium, nutrients of concern, occur in much higher concentrations in the whole-wheat flour on a 100-gram basis (percent). The fortification nutrients—thiamin, riboflavin, niacin, and iron—are similar in concentration between the two flours, but folate, as Dietary Folate Equivalent (DFE), µg, is higher in the enriched white flour.

	100 Percent Whole-Grain Wheat Flour	Enriched, Bleached, All-Purpose White Flour
Calories, kcal	339.0	364.0
Dietary fiber, g	12.2	2.7
Calcium, mg	34.0	15.0
Magnesium, mg	138.0	22.0
Potassium, mg	405.0	107.0
Folate, DFE, µg	44.0	291.0
Thiamin, mg	0.5	0.8
Riboflavin, mg	0.2	0.5
Niacin, mg	6.4	5.9
Iron, mg	3.9	4.6

Source: Agricultural Research Service Nutrient Database for Standard Reference, Release 17.

TABLE 7. Whole Grains Available in the United States

Whole grains that are consumed in the United States either as a single food (e.g., wild rice, popcorn) or as an ingredient in a multi-ingredient food (e.g., in multi-grain breads). This listing of whole grains was determined from a breakdown of foods reported consumed in nationwide food consumption surveys, by amount consumed. The foods are listed in approximate order of amount consumed, but the order may change over time. In addition, other whole grains may be consumed that are not yet represented in the surveys.

Whole wheat
Whole oats/oatmeal
Whole-grain corn
Popcorn
Brown rice
Whole rye
Whole-grain barley
Wild rice
Buckwheat
Triticale
Bulgur (cracked wheat)
Millet
Quinoa
Sorghum

Source: Agriculture Research Service Database for CSFII 1994–1996.

Fats

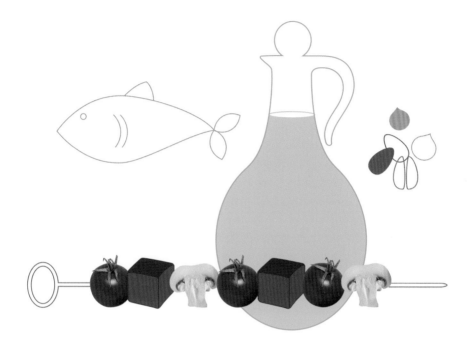

OVERVIEW

Fats and oils are part of a healthful diet, but the type of fat makes a difference to heart health, and the total amount of fat consumed is also important. High intake of saturated fats, *trans* fats, and cholesterol increases the risk of unhealthy blood lipid levels, which, in turn, may increase the risk of coronary heart disease. A high intake of fat (greater than 35 percent of calories) generally increases saturated fat intake and makes it more difficult to avoid consuming excess calories. A low intake of fats and oils (less than 20 percent of calories) increases the risk of inadequate intakes of vitamin E and of essential fatty acids and may contribute to unfavorable changes in high-density lipoprotein (HDL) blood cholesterol and triglycerides.

DISCUSSION

Fats supply energy and essential fatty acids and serve as a carrier for the absorption of the fat-soluble vitamins A, D, E, and K and carotenoids. Fats serve as building blocks of membranes and play a key regulatory role in numerous biological functions. Dietary fat is found in foods derived from both plants and animals. The recommended total fat intake is between 20 and 35 percent of calories for adults. A fat intake of 30 to 35 percent of calories is recommended for children 2 to 3 years of age and 25 to 35 percent of calories for children and adolescents 4 to 18 years of age. Few Americans consume less than 20 percent of calories from fat. Fat intakes that exceed 35 percent of calories are associated with both total increased saturated fat and calorie intakes.

To decrease their risk of elevated low-density lipoprotein (LDL) cholesterol in the blood, most Americans need to decrease their intakes of saturated fat and *trans* fats, and many need to decrease their dietary intake of cholesterol. Because men tend to have higher intakes of dietary cholesterol, it is especially important for them to meet this recommendation. Population-based studies of American diets show that intake of saturated fat is more excessive than intake of *trans* fats and cholesterol. Therefore, it is most important for Americans to decrease their intake of saturated fat. However, intake of all three should be decreased to meet recommendations. Table 8 (page 293) shows, for selected calorie levels, the maximum gram amounts of saturated fat to consume to keep saturated fat intake below 10 percent of total calorie intake. This table may be useful when combined with label-reading guidance. Table 9 (page 294) gives a few practical examples of the differences in the saturated fat content of different forms of commonly consumed foods. Table 10 (page 295) provides the major dietary sources of saturated fats in the U.S. diet listed in decreasing order. Diets can be planned to meet nutrient recommendations for linoleic acid and α-linolenic acid while providing very low amounts of saturated fatty acids.

Based on 1994–1996 data, the estimated average daily intake of *trans* fats in the United States was about 2.6 percent of total energy intake. Processed foods and oils provide approximately 80 percent of *trans* fats in the diet, compared to 20 percent that occur naturally in food from animal sources. Table 11 (page 296) provides the major dietary sources of *trans* fats listed in decreasing order. *Trans* fat content of certain processed foods has changed and is likely to continue to change as the industry reformulates products. Because the *trans* fatty acids produced in the partial hydrogenation of vegetable oils account for more than 80 percent of total intake, the food industry has an important role in decreasing *trans* fatty acid content of the food supply. Limited consumption of foods made with processed sources of *trans* fats provides the most effective means of reducing intake of *trans* fats. By looking at the food label, consumers can select products that are lowest in saturated fat, *trans* fats,[13] and cholesterol.

---

[13] Including the amount of *trans* fats on the Nutrition Facts Panel is voluntary until January 2006.

To meet the total fat recommendation of 20 to 35 percent of calories, most dietary fats should come from sources of polyunsaturated and monounsaturated fatty acids. Sources of omega-6 polyunsaturated fatty acids are liquid vegetable oils, including soybean oil, corn oil, and safflower oil. Plant sources of omega-3 polyunsaturated fatty acids (α-linolenic acid) include soybean oil, canola oil, walnuts, and flaxseed. Eicosapentaenoic acid (EPA) and docosahexaenoic acid (DHA) are omega-3 fatty acids that are contained in fish and shellfish. Fish that naturally contain more oil (e.g., salmon, trout, herring) are higher in EPA and DHA than are lean fish (e.g., cod, haddock, catfish). Limited evidence suggests an association between consumption of fatty acids in fish and reduced risks of mortality from cardiovascular disease for the general population. Other sources of EPA and DHA may provide similar benefits; however, more research is needed. Plant sources that are rich in monounsaturated fatty acids include vegetable oils (e.g., canola, olive, high oleic safflower, and sunflower oils) that are liquid at room temperature and nuts.

KEY RECOMMENDATIONS

- Consume less than 10 percent of calories from saturated fatty acids and less than 300 mg/day of cholesterol, and keep *trans* fatty acid consumption as low as possible.
- Keep total fat intake between 20 to 35 percent of calories, with most fats coming from sources of polyunsaturated and monounsaturated fatty acids, such as fish, nuts, and vegetable oils.
- When selecting and preparing meat, poultry, dry beans, and milk or milk products, make choices that are lean, low-fat, or fat-free.
- Limit intake of fats and oils high in saturated and/or *trans* fatty acids, and choose products low in such fats and oils.

Key Recommendations for Specific Population Groups

- *Children and adolescents.* Keep total fat intake between 30 to 35 percent of calories for children 2 to 3 years of age and between 25 to 35 percent of calories for children and adolescents 4 to 18 years of age, with most fats coming from sources of polyunsaturated and monounsaturated fatty acids, such as fish, nuts, and vegetable oils.

Considerations for Specific Population Groups

Evidence suggests that consuming approximately two servings of fish per week (approximately 8 ounces total) may reduce the risk of mortality from coronary heart disease and that consuming EPA and DHA may reduce the risk of mortality from cardiovascular disease in people who have already experienced a cardiac event.

Federal and State advisories provide current information about lowering exposure to environmental contaminants in fish. For example, methylmercury is a heavy metal toxin found in varying levels in nearly all fish and shellfish. For most people, the risk from mercury by eating fish and shellfish is not a health concern. However, some fish contain higher levels of mercury that may harm an unborn baby or young child's developing nervous system. The risks from mercury in fish and shellfish depend on the amount of fish eaten and the levels of mercury in the fish. Therefore, the Food and Drug Administration (FDA) and the Environmental Protection Agency are advising women of childbearing age who may become pregnant, pregnant women, nursing mothers, and young children to avoid some types of fish and shellfish and eat fish and shellfish that are lower in mercury. For more information, call FDA's food information line toll-free at 1-888-SAFEFOOD or visit http://www.cfsan.fda.gov/~dms/admehg3.html.

Lower intakes (less than 7 percent of calories from saturated fat and less than 200 mg/day of cholesterol) are recommended as part of a therapeutic diet for adults with elevated LDL blood cholesterol (i.e., above their LDL blood cholesterol goal [see table 12, page 297]). People with an elevated LDL blood cholesterol level should be under the care of a healthcare provider.

…most Americans need to decrease their intakes of saturated fat and *trans* fats, and many need to decrease their dietary intake of cholesterol.

TABLE 8. Maximum Daily Amounts of Saturated Fat To Keep Saturated Fat Below 10 Percent of Total Calorie Intake

The maximum gram amounts of saturated fat that can be consumed to keep saturated fat intake below 10 percent of total calorie intake for selected calorie levels. A 2,000-calorie example is included for consistency with the food label. This table may be useful when combined with label-reading guidance.

Total Calorie Intake	Limit on Saturated Fat Intake
1,600	18 g or less
2,000[a]	20 g or less
2,200	24 g or less
2,500[a]	25 g or less
2,800	31 g or less

[a] Percent Daily Values on the Nutrition Facts Panel of food labels are based on a 2,000-calorie diet. Values for 2,000 and 2,500 calories are rounded to the nearest 5 grams to be consistent with the Nutrition Facts Panel.

TABLE 9. Differences in Saturated Fat and Calorie Content of Commonly Consumed Foods

This table shows a few practical examples of the differences in the saturated fat content of different forms of commonly consumed foods. Comparisons are made between foods in the same food group (e.g., regular cheddar cheese and low-fat cheddar cheese), illustrating that lower saturated fat choices can be made within the same food group.

Note: Table updated to reflect 2005 DASH Eating Plan.

Food Category	Portion	Saturated Fat Content (grams)	Calories
Cheese			
• Regular cheddar cheese	1 oz	6.0	114
• Low-fat cheddar cheese	1 oz	1.2	49
Ground beef			
• Regular ground beef (25% fat)	3 oz (cooked)	6.1	236
• Extra lean ground beef (5% fat)	3 oz (cooked)	2.6	148
Milk			
• Whole milk (3.25%)	1 cup	4.6	146
• Low-fat (1%) milk	1 cup	1.5	102
Breads			
• Croissant (med)	1 medium	6.6	231
• Bagel, oat bran (4")	1 medium	0.2	227
Frozen desserts			
• Regular ice cream	½ cup	4.9	145
• Frozen yogurt, low-fat	½ cup	2.0	110
Table spreads			
• Butter	1 tsp	2.4	34
• Soft margarine with zero *trans* fats	1 tsp	0.7	25
Chicken			
• Fried chicken (leg with skin)	3 oz (cooked)	3.3	212
• Roasted chicken (breast no skin)	3 oz (cooked)	0.9	140
Fish			
• Fried fish	3 oz	2.8	195
• Baked fish	3 oz	1.5	129

Source: ARS Nutrient Database for Standard Reference, Release 17.

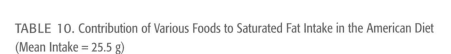
TABLE 10. Contribution of Various Foods to Saturated Fat Intake in the American Diet (Mean Intake = 25.5 g)

The major dietary sources of saturated fats in the U.S. diet listed in decreasing order.

Food Group	Contribution (percent of total sat fat consumed)
Cheese	13.1
Beef	11.7
Milk[a]	7.8
Oils	4.9
Ice cream/sherbet/frozen yogurt	4.7
Cakes/cookies/quick breads/doughnuts	4.7
Butter	4.6
Other fats[b]	4.4
Salad dressings/mayonnaise	3.7
Poultry	3.6
Margarine	3.2
Sausage	3.1
Potato chips/corn chips/popcorn	2.9
Yeast bread	2.6
Eggs	2.3

[a] The milk category includes all milk, including whole milk, low-fat milk, and fat-free milk.

[b] Shortening and animal fats.

Source: Adapted from Cotton PA, Subar AF, Friday JE, Cook A, Dietary Sources of Nutrients among U.S. Adults, 1994–1996. *JADA* 104:921-931, 2004.

TABLE 11. Contribution of Various Foods to *Trans* Fat Intake in the American Diet (Mean Intake = 5.84 g)

The major dietary sources of *trans* fats listed in decreasing order. Processed foods and oils provide approximately 80 percent of *trans* fats in the diet, compared to 20 percent that occur naturally in food from animal sources. *Trans* fats content of certain processed foods has changed and is likely to continue to change as the industry reformulates products.

Food Group	Contribution (percent of total *trans* fats consumed)
Cakes, cookies, crackers, pies, bread, etc.	40
Animal products	21
Margarine	17
Fried potatoes	8
Potato chips, corn chips, popcorn	5
Household shortening	4
Other[a]	5

[a] Includes breakfast cereal and candy. USDA analysis reported 0 grams of *trans* fats in salad dressing.

Source: Adapted from *Federal Register* notice. *Food Labeling; Trans Fatty Acids in Nutrition Labeling; Consumer Research To Consider Nutrient Content and Health Claims and Possible Footnote or Disclosure Statements; Final Rule and Proposed Rule*. Vol. 68, No. 133, p. 41433-41506, July 11, 2003. Data collected 1994-1996.

TABLE 12. Relationship Between LDL Blood Cholesterol Goal and the Level of Coronary Heart Disease Risk

Information for adults with elevated LDL blood cholesterol. LDL blood cholesterol goals for these individuals are related to the level of coronary heart disease risk. People with an elevated LDL blood cholesterol value should make therapeutic lifestyle changes (diet, physical activity, weight control) under the care of a healthcare provider to lower LDL blood cholesterol.

If Someone Has:	LDL Blood Cholesterol Goal Is:
CHD or CHD risk equivalent[a]	Less than 100 mg/dL
Two or more risk factors other than elevated LDL blood cholesterol[b]	Less than 130 mg/dL
Zero or one risk factor other than elevated LDL blood cholesterol[b]	Less than 160 mg/dL

[a] CHD (coronary heart disease) risk equivalent = presence of clinical atherosclerotic disease that confers high risk for CHD events:
 - Clinical CHD
 - Symptomatic carotid artery disease
 - Peripheral arterial disease
 - Abdominal aortic aneurysm
 - Diabetes
 - Two or more risk factors with >20% risk for CHD (or myocardial infarction or CHD death) within 10 years

[b] Major risk factors that affect your LDL goal:
 - Cigarette smoking
 - High blood pressure (140/90 mmHg or higher or on blood pressure medication)
 - Low HDL blood cholesterol (less than 40 mg/dL)
 - Family history of early heart disease (heart disease in father or brother before age 55; heart disease in mother or sister before age 65)
 - Age (men 45 years or older; women 55 years or older)

Source: NIH Publication No. 01-3290, U.S. Department of Health and Human Services, National Institutes of Health, National Heart, Lung, and Blood Institute, National Cholesterol Education Program Brochure, High Blood Cholesterol - What You Need to Know, May 2001. http://www.nhlbi.nih.gov/health/public/heart/chol/hbc_what.htm.

Carbohydrates

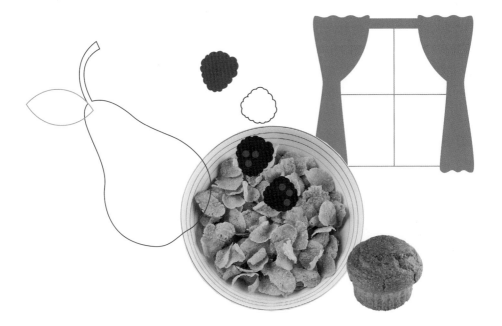

OVERVIEW

Carbohydrates are part of a healthful diet. The AMDR for carbohydrates is 45 to 65 percent of total calories. Dietary fiber is composed of nondigestible carbohydrates and lignin intrinsic and intact in plants. Diets rich in dietary fiber have been shown to have a number of beneficial effects, including decreased risk of coronary heart disease and improvement in laxation. There is also interest in the potential relationship between diets containing fiber-rich foods and lower risk of type 2 diabetes. Sugars and starches supply energy to the body in the form of glucose, which is the only energy source for red blood cells and is the preferred energy source for the brain, central nervous system, placenta, and fetus. Sugars can be naturally present in foods (such as the fructose in fruit or the lactose in milk) or added to the food. Added sugars, also known as caloric sweeteners, are sugars and syrups that are added to foods at the table or during processing or preparation (such as high-fructose corn syrup in sweetened beverages and baked products). Although the body's response to sugars does not depend on whether they are naturally present in a food or added to the food, added sugars supply calories but few or no nutrients.

Consequently, it is important to choose carbohydrates wisely. Foods in the basic food groups that provide carbohydrates—fruits, vegetables, grains, and milk—are important sources of many nutrients. Choosing plenty of these foods, within the context of a calorie-controlled diet, can promote health and reduce chronic disease risk. However, the greater the consumption of foods containing large amounts of added sugars, the more difficult it is to consume enough nutrients without gaining weight. Consumption of added sugars provides calories while providing little, if any, of the essential nutrients.

DISCUSSION

The recommended dietary fiber intake is 14 grams per 1,000 calories consumed. Initially, some Americans will find it challenging to achieve this level of intake. However, making fiber-rich food choices more often will move people toward this goal and is likely to confer significant health benefits.

The majority of servings from the fruit group should come from whole fruit (fresh, frozen, canned, dried) rather than juice. Increasing the proportion of fruit that is eaten in the form of whole fruit rather than juice is desirable to increase fiber intake. However, inclusion of some juice, such as orange juice, can help meet recommended levels of potassium intake. Appendixes B-1 and B-8 list some of the best sources of potassium and dietary fiber, respectively.

Legumes—such as dry beans and peas—are especially rich in fiber and should be consumed several times per week. They are considered part of both the vegetable group and the meat and beans group as they contain nutrients found in each of these food groups.

Diets rich in dietary fiber
have been shown to have
a number of beneficial effects.

KEY RECOMMENDATIONS

- Choose fiber-rich fruits, vegetables, and whole grains often.
- Choose and prepare foods and beverages with little added sugars or caloric sweeteners, such as amounts suggested by the USDA Food Guide and the DASH Eating Plan.
- Reduce the incidence of dental caries by practicing good oral hygiene and consuming sugar- and starch-containing foods and beverages less frequently.

Consuming at least half the recommended grain servings as whole grains is important, for all ages, at each calorie level, to meet the fiber recommendation. Consuming at least 3 ounce-equivalents of whole grains per day can reduce the risk of coronary heart disease, may help with weight maintenance, and may lower risk for other chronic diseases. Thus, at lower calorie levels, adults should consume more than half (specifically, at least 3 ounce-equivalents) of whole grains per day, by substituting whole grains for refined grains. (See table 7, page 288, for a list of whole grains available in the United States.)

Individuals who consume food or beverages high in added sugars tend to consume more calories than those who consume food or beverages low in added sugars; they also tend to consume lower amounts of micronutrients. Although more research is needed, available prospective studies show a positive association between the consumption of calorically sweetened beverages and weight gain. For this reason, decreased intake of such foods, especially beverages with caloric sweeteners, is recommended to reduce calorie intake and help achieve recommended nutrient intakes and weight control.

Total discretionary calories should not exceed the allowance for any given calorie level, as shown in the USDA Food Guide (see Nutrient Adequacy, pages 257 to 268). The discretionary calorie allowance covers all calories from added sugars, alcohol, and the additional fat found in even moderate fat choices from the milk and meat group. For example, the 2,000-calorie pattern includes only about 267 discretionary calories. At 29 percent of calories from total fat (including 18 g of solid fat), if no alcohol is consumed, then only 8 teaspoons (32 g) of added sugars can be afforded. This is less than the amount in a typical 12-ounce calorically sweetened soft drink. If fat is decreased to 22 percent of calories, then 18 teaspoons (72 g) of added sugars is allowed. If fat is increased to 35 percent of calories, then no allowance remains for added sugars, even if alcohol is not consumed.

In some cases, small amounts of sugars added to nutrient-dense foods, such as breakfast cereals and reduced-fat milk products, may increase a person's intake of such foods by enhancing the palatability of these products, thus improving nutrient intake without contributing excessive calories. The major sources of added sugars are listed in table 13, page 304 (app. A-3 provides examples of how added sugars can fit into the discretionary calorie allowance).

The Nutrition Facts Panel on the food label provides the amount of total sugars but does not list added sugars separately. People should examine the ingredient list to find out whether a food contains added sugars. The ingredient list is usually located under the Nutrition Facts Panel or on the side of a food label. Ingredients are listed in order of predominance, by weight; that is, the ingredient with the greatest contribution to the product weight is listed first and the ingredient contributing the least amount is listed last. Table 14 (page 304) lists ingredients that are included in the term "added sugars."[14]

...the greater the consumption of foods containing large amounts of added sugars, the more difficult it is to consume enough nutrients without gaining weight.

Sugars and starches contribute to dental caries by providing substrate for bacterial fermentation in the mouth. Thus, the frequency and duration of consumption of starches and sugars can be important factors because they increase exposure to cariogenic substrates. Drinking fluoridated water and/or using fluoride-containing dental hygiene products help reduce the risk of dental caries. Most bottled water is not fluoridated. With the increase in consumption of bottled water, there is concern that Americans may not be getting enough fluoride for maintenance of oral health. A combined approach of reducing the frequency and duration of exposure to fermentable carbohydrate intake and optimizing oral hygiene practices, such as drinking fluori-

---

[14] For information on amounts of added sugars in some common foods, see Krebs-Smith, SM. Choose beverages and foods to moderate your intake of sugars: measurement requires quantification. *The Journal of Nutrition (J Nutr)* 131(2S-I): 527S-535S, 2001.

dated water and brushing and flossing teeth, is the most effective way to reduce incidence of dental caries.

Considerations for Specific Population Groups

Older Adults

Dietary fiber is important for laxation. Since constipation may affect up to 20 percent of people over 65 years of age, older adults should choose to consume foods rich in dietary fiber. Other causes of constipation among this age group may include drug interactions with laxation and lack of appropriate hydration (see Nutrient Adequacy, pages 257 to 268).

Children

Carbohydrate intakes of children need special considerations with regard to obtaining sufficient amounts of fiber, avoiding excessive amounts of calories from added sugars, and preventing dental caries. Several cross-sectional surveys on U.S. children and adolescents have found inadequate dietary fiber intakes, which could be improved by increasing consumption of whole fruits, vegetables, and whole-grain products. Sugars can improve the palatability of foods and beverages that otherwise might not be consumed. This may explain why the consumption of sweetened dairy foods and beverages and presweetened cereals is positively associated with children's and adolescents' nutrient intake. However, beverages with caloric sweeteners, sugars and sweets, and other sweetened foods that provide little or no nutrients are negatively associated with diet quality and can contribute to excessive energy intakes, affirming the importance of reducing added sugar intake substantially from current levels. Most of the studies of preschool children suggest a positive association between sucrose consumption and dental caries, though other factors (particularly infrequent brushing or not using fluoridated toothpaste) are more predictive of caries outcome than is sugar consumption.

TABLE 13. Major Sources of Added Sugars (Caloric Sweeteners) in the American Diet

Food groups that contribute more than 5 percent of the added sugars to the American diet in decreasing order.

Food Categories	Contribution to Added Sugars Intake (percent of total added sugars consumed)
Regular soft drinks	33.0
Sugars and candy	16.1
Cakes, cookies, pies	12.9
Fruit drinks (fruitades and fruit punch)	9.7
Dairy desserts and milk products (ice cream, sweetened yogurt, and sweetened milk)	8.6
Other grains (cinnamon toast and honey-nut waffles)	5.8

Source: Guthrie and Morton, *Journal of the American Dietetic Association*, 2000.

TABLE 14. Names for Added Sugars That Appear on Food Labels

Some of the names for added sugars that may be in processed foods and listed on the label ingredients list.

Brown sugar	Invert sugar
Corn sweetener	Lactose
Corn syrup	Maltose
Dextrose	Malt syrup
Fructose	Molasses
Fruit juice concentrates	Raw sugar
Glucose	Sucrose
High-fructose corn syrup	Sugar
Honey	Syrup

Sodium and Potassium

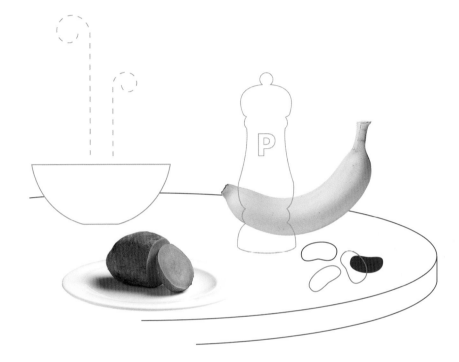

OVERVIEW

On average, the higher an individual's salt (sodium chloride) intake, the higher an individual's blood pressure. Nearly all Americans consume substantially more salt than they need. Decreasing salt intake is advisable to reduce the risk of elevated blood pressure. Keeping blood pressure in the normal range reduces an individual's risk of coronary heart disease, stroke, congestive heart failure, and kidney disease. Many American adults will develop hypertension (high blood pressure) during their lifetime. Lifestyle changes can prevent or delay the onset of high blood pressure and can lower elevated blood pressure. These changes include reducing salt intake, increasing potassium intake, losing excess body weight, increasing physical activity, and eating an overall healthful diet.

DISCUSSION

Salt is sodium chloride. Food labels list sodium rather than salt content. When reading a Nutrition Facts Panel on a food product, look for the sodium content. Foods that are low in sodium (less than 140 mg or 5 percent of the Daily Value [DV]) are low in salt.

Common sources of sodium found in the food supply are provided in figure 4 (page 308). On average, the natural salt content of food accounts for only about 10 percent of total intake, while discretionary salt use (i.e., salt added at the table or while cooking) provides another 5 to 10 percent of total intake. Approximately 75 percent is derived from salt added by manufacturers. In addition, foods served by food establishments may be high in sodium. It is important to read the food label and determine the sodium content of food, which can vary by several hundreds of milligrams in similar foods. For example, the sodium content in regular tomato soup may be 700 mg per cup in one brand and 1,100 mg per cup in another brand. Reading labels, comparing sodium contents of foods, and purchasing the lower sodium brand may be one strategy to lower total sodium intake (see table 15, page 308, for examples of these foods).

An individual's preference for salt is not fixed. After consuming foods lower in salt for a period of time, taste for salt tends to decrease. Use of other flavorings may satisfy an individual's taste. While salt substitutes containing potassium chloride may be useful for some individuals, they can be harmful to people with certain medical conditions. These individuals should consult a healthcare provider before trying salt substitutes.

Lifestyle changes can prevent or delay the onset of high blood pressure and can lower elevated blood pressure.

Discretionary salt use is fairly stable, even when foods offered are lower in sodium than typical foods consumed. When consumers are offered a lower sodium product, they typically do not add table salt to compensate for the lower sodium content, even when available. Therefore, any program for reducing the salt consumption of a population should concentrate primarily on reducing the salt used during food processing and on changes in food selection (e.g., more fresh, less-processed items, less sodium-dense foods) and preparation.

Reducing salt intake is one of several ways that people may lower their blood pressure. The relationship between salt intake and blood pressure is direct and progressive without an apparent threshold. On average, the higher a person's salt intake, the higher the blood pressure. Reducing blood pressure, ideally to the normal range, reduces the risk of stroke, heart disease, heart failure, and kidney disease.

KEY RECOMMENDATIONS

- Consume less than 2,300 mg (approximately 1 tsp of salt) of sodium per day.
- Choose and prepare foods with little salt. At the same time, consume potassium-rich foods, such as fruits and vegetables.

Key Recommendations for Specific Population Groups

- *Individuals with hypertension, blacks, and middle-aged and older adults.* Aim to consume no more than 1,500 mg of sodium per day, and meet the potassium recommendation (4,700 mg/day) with food.

Another dietary measure to lower blood pressure is to consume a diet rich in potassium. A potassium-rich diet also blunts the effects of salt on blood pressure, may reduce the risk of developing kidney stones, and possibly decrease bone loss with age. The recommended intake of potassium for adolescents and adults is 4,700 mg/day. Recommended intakes for potassium for children 1 to 3 years of age is 3,000 mg/day, 4 to 8 years of age is 3,800 mg/day, and 9 to 13 years of age is 4,500 mg/day. Potassium should come from food sources. Fruits and vegetables, which are rich in potassium with its bicarbonate precursors, favorably affect acid-base metabolism, which may reduce risk of kidney stones and bone loss. Potassium-rich fruits and vegetables include leafy green vegetables, fruit from vines, and root vegetables. Meat, milk, and cereal products also contain potassium, but may not have the same effect on acid-base metabolism. Dietary sources of potassium are listed in table 5 (page 286) and appendix B-1.

Considerations for Specific Population Groups

Individuals With Hypertension, Blacks, and Middle-Aged and Older Adults. Some individuals tend to be more salt sensitive than others, including people with hypertension, blacks, and middle-aged and older adults. Because blacks commonly have a relatively low intake of potassium and a high prevalence of elevated blood pressure and salt sensitivity, this population subgroup may especially benefit from an increased dietary intake of potassium. Dietary potassium can lower blood pressure and blunt the effects of salt on blood pressure in some individuals. While salt substitutes containing potassium chloride may be useful for some individuals, they can be harmful to people with certain medical conditions. These individuals should consult a healthcare provider before using salt substitutes.

FIGURE 4. Sources of Dietary Sodium

The relative amounts of dietary sodium in the American diet.

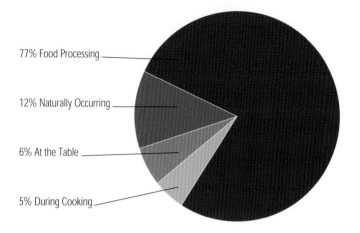

77% Food Processing

12% Naturally Occurring

6% At the Table

5% During Cooking

Source: Mattes RD, Donnelly D. Relative contributions of dietary sodium sources. *J Am Coll Nutr.* 1991 Aug;10(4):383-393.

TABLE 15. Range of Sodium Content for Selected Foods

The ranges of sodium content for selected foods available in the retail market. This table is provided to exemplify the importance of reading the food label to determine the sodium content of food, which can vary by several hundreds of milligrams in similar foods.

Food Group	Serving Size	Range (mg)
Breads, all types	1 oz	95–210
Frozen pizza, plain, cheese	4 oz	450–1200
Frozen vegetables, all types	½ c	2–160
Salad dressing, regular fat, all types	2 Tbsp	110–505
Salsa	2 Tbsp	150–240
Soup (tomato), reconstituted	8 oz	700–1260
Tomato juice	8 oz (~1 c)	340–1040
Potato chips[a]	1 oz (28.4 g)	120–180
Tortilla chips[a]	1 oz (28.4 g)	105–160
Pretzels[a]	1 oz (28.4 g)	290–560

[a] All snack foods are regular flavor, salted.

Source: Agricultural Research Service Nutrient Database for Standard Reference, Release 17 and recent manufacturers label data from retail market surveys. Serving sizes were standardized to be comparable among brands within a food. Pizza and bread slices vary in size and weight across brands.

Note: None of the examples provided were labeled low-sodium products.

Alcoholic Beverages

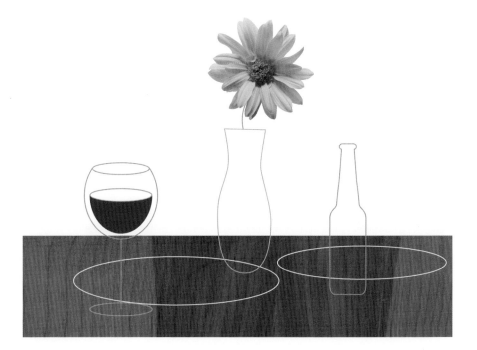

OVERVIEW

The consumption of alcohol can have beneficial or harmful effects depending on the amount consumed, age and other characteristics of the person consuming the alcohol, and specifics of the situation. In 2002, 55 percent of U.S. adults were current drinkers. Forty-five percent of U.S. adults do not drink any alcohol at all.[15] Abstention is an important option. Fewer Americans consume alcohol today as compared to 50 to 100 years ago.

The hazards of heavy alcohol consumption are well known and include increased risk of liver cirrhosis, hypertension, cancers of the upper gastrointestinal tract, injury, violence, and death. Moreover, certain individuals who are more susceptible to the harmful effects of alcohol should not drink at all. In addition, alcohol should be avoided by those participating in activities that require attention, skill, and/or coordination.

[15] Behavioral Risk Factor Surveillance System, Surveillance for Certain Health Behaviors Among Selected Local Areas–United States, Behavioral Risk Factor Surveillance System, 2002, *MMWR*, 53, No SS-05. http://www.cdc.gov/brfss/.

Alcohol may have beneficial effects when consumed in moderation. The lowest all-cause mortality occurs at an intake of one to two drinks per day. The lowest coronary heart disease mortality also occurs at an intake of one to two drinks per day. Morbidity and mortality are highest among those drinking large amounts of alcohol.

DISCUSSION

Alcoholic beverages supply calories but few essential nutrients (see table 16, page 312). As a result, excessive alcohol consumption makes it difficult to ingest sufficient nutrients within an individual's daily calorie allotment and to maintain a healthy weight. Although the consumption of one to two alcoholic beverages per day is not associated with macronutrient or micronutrient deficiencies or with overall dietary quality, heavy drinkers may be at risk of malnutrition if the calories derived from alcohol are substituted for those in nutritious foods.

The majority of American adults consume alcohol. Those who do so should drink alcoholic beverages in moderation. Moderation is defined as the consumption of up to one drink per day for women and up to two drinks per day for men. Twelve fluid ounces of regular beer, 5 fluid ounces of wine, or 1.5 fluid ounces of 80-proof distilled spirits count as one drink for purposes of explaining moderation. This definition of moderation is not intended as an average over several days but rather as the amount consumed on any single day.

Alcoholic beverages supply calories but few essential nutrients.

The effect of alcohol consumption varies depending on the amount consumed and an individual's characteristics and circumstances. Alcoholic beverages are harmful when consumed in excess. Excess alcohol consumption alters judgment and can lead to dependency or addiction and other serious health problems such as cirrhosis of the liver, inflammation of the pancreas, and damage to the heart and brain. Even less than heavy consumption of alcohol is associated with significant risks. Consuming more than one drink per day for women and two drinks per day for men increases the risk for motor vehicle accidents, other injuries, high blood pressure, stroke, violence, some types of cancer, and suicide. Compared with women who do not drink, women who consume one drink per day appear to have a slightly higher risk of breast cancer.

KEY RECOMMENDATIONS

- Those who choose to drink alcoholic beverages should do so sensibly and in moderation—defined as the consumption of up to one drink per day for women and up to two drinks per day for men.
- Alcoholic beverages should not be consumed by some individuals, including those who cannot restrict their alcohol intake, women of childbearing age who may become pregnant, pregnant and lactating women, children and adolescents, individuals taking medications that can interact with alcohol, and those with specific medical conditions.
- Alcoholic beverages should be avoided by individuals engaging in activities that require attention, skill, or coordination, such as driving or operating machinery.

Studies suggest adverse effects even at moderate alcohol consumption levels in specific situations and individuals. Individuals in some situations should avoid alcohol—those who plan to drive, operate machinery, or take part in other activities that require attention, skill, or coordination. Some people, including children and adolescents, women of childbearing age who may become pregnant, pregnant and lactating women, individuals who cannot restrict alcohol intake, individuals taking medications that can interact with alcohol, and individuals with specific medical conditions should not drink at all. Even moderate drinking during pregnancy may have behavioral or developmental consequences for the baby. Heavy drinking during pregnancy can produce a range of behavioral and psychosocial problems, malformation, and mental retardation in the baby.

Moderate alcohol consumption may have beneficial health effects in some individuals. In middle-aged and older adults, a daily intake of one to two alcoholic beverages per day is associated with the lowest all-cause mortality. More specifically, compared to non-drinkers, adults who consume one to two alcoholic beverages a day appear to have a lower risk of coronary heart disease. In contrast, among younger adults alcohol consumption appears to provide little, if any, health benefit, and alcohol use among young adults is associated with a higher risk of traumatic injury and death. As noted previously, a number of strategies reduce the risk of chronic disease, including a healthful diet, physical activity, avoidance of smoking, and maintenance of a healthy weight. Furthermore, it is not recommended that anyone begin drinking or drink more frequently on the basis of health considerations.

TABLE 16. Calories in Selected Alcoholic Beverages

This table is a guide to estimate the caloric intake from various alcoholic beverages. An example serving volume and the calories in that drink are shown for beer, wine, and distilled spirits. Higher alcohol content (higher percent alcohol or higher proof) and mixing alcohol with other beverages, such as calorically sweetened soft drinks, tonic water, fruit juice, or cream, increases the amount of calories in the beverage. Alcoholic beverages supply calories but provide few essential nutrients.

Beverage	Approximate Calories Per 1 Fluid Oz[a]	Example Serving Volume	Approximate Total Calories[b]
Beer (regular)	12	12 oz	144
Beer (light)	9	12 oz	108
White wine	20	5 oz	100
Red wine	21	5 oz	105
Sweet dessert wine	47	3 oz	141
80-proof distilled spirits (gin, rum, vodka, whiskey)	64	1.5 oz	96

[a] Source: Agricultural Research Service (ARS) Nutrient Database for Standard Reference (SR), Release 17. (http://www.nal.usda.gov/fnic/foodcomp/index.html) Calories are calculated to the nearest whole number per 1 fluid oz.

[b] The total calories and alcohol content vary depending on the brand. Moreover, adding mixers to an alcoholic beverage can contribute calories in addition to the calories from the alcohol itself.

Food Safety

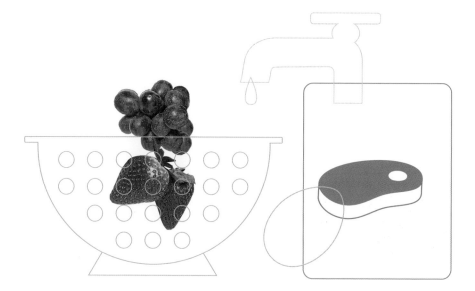

OVERVIEW

Avoiding foods contaminated with harmful bacteria, viruses, parasites, toxins, and chemical and physical contaminants is vital for healthful eating. The signs and symptoms of foodborne illness range from gastrointestinal symptoms, such as upset stomach, diarrhea, fever, vomiting, abdominal cramps, and dehydration, to more severe systemic illness, such as paralysis and meningitis. It is estimated that every year about 76 million people in the United States become ill from pathogens in food; of these, about 5,000 die. Consumers can take simple measures to reduce their risk of foodborne illness, especially in the home.

DISCUSSION

The most important food safety problem is microbial foodborne illness. All those who handle food, including farmers, food producers, individuals who work in markets and food service establishments, and other food preparers, have a responsibility to keep food as safe as possible. To keep food safe, people who prepare food should clean hands, food contact surfaces, and fruits and vegetables; separate raw, cooked, and ready-to-eat foods; cook foods to a safe internal temperature; chill perishable food promptly; and defrost food properly. For more important information on cooking, cleaning, separating, and chilling, see www.fightbac.org.

Consumers can take simple measures to reduce their risk of foodborne illness, especially in the home.

When preparing and consuming food, it is essential to wash hands often, particularly before and after preparing food, especially after handling raw meat, poultry, eggs, or seafood. A good hand washing protocol includes wetting hands; applying soap; rubbing hands vigorously together for 20 seconds; rinsing hands thoroughly under clean, running warm water; and drying hands completely using a clean disposable or cloth towel.

Washing may be the only method that consumers have to reduce pathogen load on fresh produce that will not be either peeled or subsequently cooked. A good protocol for washing fresh fruits and vegetables includes removing and discarding outer leaves, washing produce just before cooking or eating, washing under running potable water, scrubbing with a clean brush or with hands, and drying the fruits or vegetables using a clean disposable or cloth towel. Free moisture on produce may promote survival and growth of microbial populations. Therefore, drying the food is critical if the item will not be eaten or cooked right away.

People should read the labels of bagged produce to determine if it is ready-to-eat. Ready-to-eat, prewashed bagged produce can be used without further washing if kept refrigerated and used by the "use-by" date. If desired, prewashed, ready-to-eat produce can be washed again.

Raw meat and poultry should not be washed because this creates the danger of cross-contamination and is not necessary. Washing these foods can allow most bacteria that are present on the surface of the meat or poultry to spread to ready-to-eat foods, kitchen utensils, and counter surfaces.

It is important to separate raw, cooked, and ready-to-eat foods while shopping, preparing, or storing foods. This prevents cross-contamination from one food to another. In addition, refrigerator surfaces can become contaminated from high-risk foods such as raw meats, poultry, fish, uncooked hot dogs, certain deli meats, or raw vegetables. If not cleaned, contaminated refrigerator surfaces can, in turn, serve as a vehicle for contaminating other foods.

Uncooked and undercooked meat, poultry, and eggs and egg products are potentially unsafe. Raw meat, poultry, and eggs should always be cooked to a safe internal temperature (see fig. 5, page 317). The best way to tell if meat, poultry, and egg dishes are cooked safely is to use a food thermometer. Leftover refrigerator foods should also be reheated to the proper internal temperature. Bacteria grow most rapidly in the range of 40°F and 140°F. To keep food out of this danger zone, keep cold food cold (below 40°F) and hot food hot (above 140°F). Figure 5 provides information for temperature rules for proper cooking and food handling. Proper cooking makes most uncooked foods safe.

KEY RECOMMENDATIONS

- To avoid microbial foodborne illness:
  - Clean hands, food contact surfaces, and fruits and vegetables. Meat and poultry should *not* be washed or rinsed.
  - Separate raw, cooked, and ready-to-eat foods while shopping, preparing, or storing foods.
  - Cook foods to a safe temperature to kill microorganisms.
  - Chill (refrigerate) perishable food promptly and defrost foods properly.
  - Avoid raw (unpasteurized) milk or any products made from unpasteurized milk, raw or partially cooked eggs or foods containing raw eggs, raw or undercooked meat and poultry, unpasteurized juices, and raw sprouts.

Key Recommendations for Specific Population Groups
- *Infants and young children, pregnant women, older adults, and those who are immunocompromised.* Do not eat or drink raw (unpasteurized) milk or any products made from unpasteurized milk, raw or partially cooked eggs or foods containing raw eggs, raw or undercooked meat and poultry, raw or undercooked fish or shellfish, unpasteurized juices, and raw sprouts.
- *Pregnant women, older adults, and those who are immunocompromised:* Only eat certain deli meats and frankfurters that have been reheated to steaming hot.

The refrigerator should be set at no higher than 40°F and the freezer at 0°F, and these temperatures should be checked with an appliance thermometer. Refrigerated leftovers may become unsafe within 3 to 4 days. Despite the appearance of a food, it may not be safe to eat. Not all bacterial growth causes a food's surface to discolor or smell bad. It may be unsafe to taste fresh or leftover food items when there is any doubt about their safety. Safe disposal of the food is indicated if there is a question about whether or not a food is safe to eat. "If in doubt—throw it out."

Considerations for Specific Population Groups

Some people may be at high risk for developing foodborne illness. These include pregnant women and their fetuses, young children, older adults, people with weakened immune systems, and individuals with certain chronic illnesses. These people should pay extra attention to food safety advice.

For example, pregnant women, older adults, and those who are immunocompromised are at risk of developing listeriosis, a potentially life-threatening illness caused by the bacterium *Listeria monocytogenes*. Some deli meats and frankfurters that have not been reheated to steaming hot and some ready-to-eat foods are associated with listeriosis and pose a high risk to certain individuals. All these foods should be heated to a safe internal temperature. In addition, these individuals should take special care not to eat or drink raw (unpasteurized) milk or any products made from unpasteurized milk (such as some soft cheeses), raw or partially cooked eggs or foods containing raw eggs, raw or undercooked meat and poultry, unpasteurized juices, and raw sprouts. They should also avoid raw or undercooked fish or shellfish.

New information on food safety is constantly emerging. Recommendations and precautions for people at high risk are updated as scientists learn more about preventing foodborne illness. Individuals in high-risk categories should seek guidance from a healthcare provider. In addition, up-to-date information is available at the Government's food safety website at www.foodsafety.gov.

FIGURE 5. Temperature Rules for Safe Cooking and Handling of Foods

Safe cooking and holding temperatures for foods. Bacteria multiply rapidly between 40°F and 140°F, doubling in number in as little as 20 minutes. To keep food out of this danger zone, keep cold food cold and hot food hot. Keep food cold in the refrigerator, in coolers, or on the service line on ice. Set your refrigerator no higher than 40°F and the freezer at 0°F. Keep hot food in the oven, in heated chafing dishes, or in preheated steam tables, warming trays, and/or slow cookers. Use a clean thermometer that measures the internal temperature of cooked food to make sure meat, poultry, and casseroles are cooked to the temperatures as indicated in the figure.

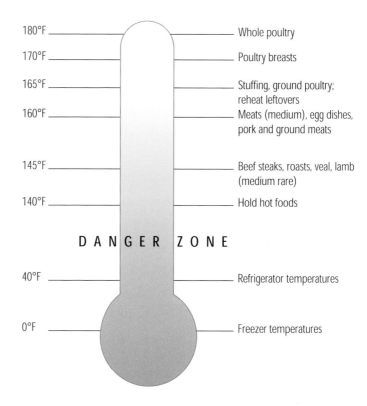

Appendixes

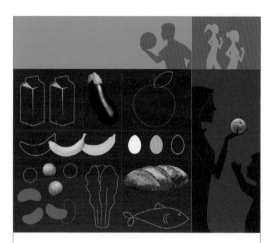

Dietary Guidelines
for Americans
2005

U.S. Department of Health and Human Services
U.S. Department of Agriculture
www.healthierus.gov/dietaryguidelines

APPENDIX A. EATING PATTERNS

Appendix A-1: The DASH Eating Plan at 1,600-, 2,000-, 2600-, and 3,100-Calorie Levels[a]

The DASH eating plan is based on 1,600, 2,000, 2,600 and 3,100 calories. The number of daily servings in a food group vary depending on caloric needs (see table 3 on page 268 to determine caloric needs). This chart can aid in planning menus and food selection in restaurants and grocery stores.

Note: Table updated to reflect 2005 DASH Eating Plan.

Food Groups	1,600 Calories	2,000 Calories	2,600 Calories	3,100 Calories	Serving Sizes	Examples and Notes	Significance of Each Food Group to the DASH Eating Plan
Grains[b]	6 servings	6–8 servings	10–11 servings	12–13 servings	1 slice bread, 1 oz dry cereal[c], 1/2 cup cooked rice, pasta, or cereal	Whole wheat bread, English muffin, pita bread, bagel, cereals, grits, oatmeal, crackers, unsalted pretzels, and popcorn	Major sources of energy and fiber
Vegetables	3–4 servings	4–5 servings	5–6 servings	6 servings	1 cup raw leafy vegetable 1/2 cup cut-up raw or cooked vegetable 1/2 cup vegetable juice	Tomatoes, potatoes, carrots, green peas, squash, broccoli, turnip greens, collards, kale, spinach, artichokes, green beans, lima beans, sweetpotatoes	Rich sources of potassium, magnesium, and fiber
Fruits	4 servings	4–5 servings	5–6 servings	6 servings	1 medium fruit 1/4 cup dried fruit 1/2 cup fresh, frozen, or canned fruit 1/2 cup fruit juice	Apricots, bananas, dates, grapes, oranges, orange juice, grapefruit, grapefruit juice, mangoes, melons, peaches, pineapples, prunes, raisins, strawberries, tangerines	Important sources of potassium, magnesium, and fiber
Fat-free or low-fat milk and milk products	2–3 servings	2–3 servings	3 servings	3–4 servings	1 cup milk 1 cup yogurt 1 1/2 oz cheese	Fat-free or low-fat milk or buttermilk, fat-free or low-fat regular or frozen yogurt, fat-free, low-fat, or reduced fat cheese	Major sources of calcium and protein

Appendix A-1 continues on page 321

Appendix A-1: Continued

Food Groups	1,600 Calories	2,000 Calories	2,600 Calories	3,100 Calories	Serving Sizes	Examples and Notes	Significance of Each Food Group to the DASH Eating Plan
Lean meats, poultry, and fish	1–2 servings	2 or less servings	2 servings	2–3 servings	3 oz cooked meats, poultry, or fish	Select only lean; trim away visible fats; broil, roast, or boil instead of frying; remove skin from poultry (1 oz meat = 1 egg[d])	Rich sources of protein and magnesium
Nuts, seeds, and legumes	3–4 servings/ week	4–5 servings/ week	1 serving	1 serving	1/3 cup or 1 1/2 oz nuts; 2 Tbsp peanut butter; 2 Tbsp or 1/2 oz seeds; 1/2 cup cooked dry beans or peas	Almonds, filberts, mixed nuts, peanuts, walnuts, sunflower seeds, kidney beans, lentils	Rich sources of energy, magnesium, potassium, protein, and fiber
Fat and oils[e]	2 servings	2–3 servings	3 servings	4 servings	1 tsp soft margarine 1 Tbsp mayonnaise 2 Tbsp salad dressing 1 tsp vegetable oil	Soft margarine, low-fat mayonnaise, light salad dressing, vegetable oil (such as olive, corn, canola, or safflower)	The DASH study had 27 percent of calories as fat (low in saturated fat), including fat in or added to foods
Sweets and added sugars	0 servings	5 or less servings/ week	2 or less servings	2 or less servings	1 Tbsp sugar 1 Tbsp jelly or jam 1/2 cup sorbet and ices 1 cup lemonade	Maple syrup, sugar, jelly, jam, fruit-flavored gelatin, hard candy, fruit punch, sorbet and ices	Sweets should be low in fat

[a] www.nhlbi.nih.gov, Karanja NM et al. *JADA* 8:S19–27, 1999.

[b] Whole grains are recommended for most grain servings to meet fiber recommendations.

[c] Equals 1/2–1 1/4 cups, depending on cereal type. Check the product's Nutrition Facts Label.

[d] Since eggs are high in cholesterol, limit egg yolk intake to no more than 4 per week; 2 egg whites have the same protein content as 1 oz of meat.

[e] Fat content changes serving counts for fats and oils: For example, 1 Tbsp of regular salad dressing equals 1 serving; 1 Tbsp of a low-fat dressing equals 1/2 serving; 1 Tbsp of a fat-free dressing equals 0 servings.

Appendix A-2. USDA Food Guide

The suggested amounts of food to consume from the basic food groups, subgroups, and oils to meet recommended nutrient intakes at 12 different calorie levels. Nutrient and energy contributions from each group are calculated according to the nutrient-dense forms of foods in each group (e.g., lean meats and fat-free milk). The table also shows the discretionary calorie allowance that can be accommodated within each calorie level, in addition to the suggested amounts of nutrient-dense forms of foods in each group.

Daily Amount of Food From Each Group (vegetable subgroup amounts are per week)						
Calorie Level	1,000	1,200	1,400	1,600	1,800	2,000
Food Group[1]	Food group amounts shown in cup (c) or ounce-equivalents (oz-eq), with number of servings (srv) in parentheses when it differs from the other units. See note for quantity equivalents for foods in each group.[2] Oils are shown in grams (g).					
Fruits	1 c (2 srv)	1 c (2 srv)	1.5 c (3 srv)	1.5 c (3 srv)	1.5 c (3 srv)	2 c (4 srv)
Vegetables[3]	1 c (2 srv)	1.5 c (3 srv)	1.5 c (3 srv)	2 c (4 srv)	2.5 c (5 srv)	2.5 c (5 srv)
Dark green veg.	1 c/wk	1.5 c/wk	1.5 c/wk	2 c/wk	3 c/wk	3 c/wk
Orange veg.	.5 c/wk	1 c/wk	1 c/wk	1.5 c/wk	2 c/wk	2 c/wk
Legumes	.5 c/wk	1 c/wk	1 c/wk	2.5 c/wk	3 c/wk	3 c/wk
Starchy veg.	1.5 c/wk	2.5 c/wk	2.5 c/wk	2.5 c/wk	3 c/wk	3 c/wk
Other veg.	3.5 c/wk	4.5 c/wk	4.5 c/wk	5.5 c/wk	6.5 c/wk	6.5 c/wk
Grains[4]	3 oz-eq	4 oz-eq	5 oz-eq	5 oz-eq	6 oz-eq	6 oz-eq
Whole grains	1.5	2	2.5	3	3	3
Other grains	1.5	2	2.5	2	3	3
Lean meat and beans	2 oz-eq	3 oz-eq	4 oz-eq	5 oz-eq	5 oz-eq	5.5 oz-eq
Milk	2 c	2 c	2 c	3 c	3 c	3 c
Oils[5]	15 g	17 g	17 g	22 g	24 g	27 g
Discretionary calorie allowance[6]	165	171	171	132	195	267

Appendix A-2 continues on page 323

Appendix A-2: Continued

Daily Amount of Food From Each Group (vegetable subgroup amounts are per week)						
Calorie Level	2,200	2,400	2,600	2,800	3,000	3,200
Food Group[1]	Food group amounts shown in cup (c) or ounce-equivalents (oz-eq), with number of servings (srv) in parentheses when it differs from the other units. See note for quantity equivalents for foods in each group.[2] Oils are shown in grams (g).					
Fruits	2 c (4 srv)	2 c (4 srv)	2 c (4 srv)	2.5 c (5 srv)	2.5 c (5 srv)	2.5 c (5 srv)
Vegetables[3]	3 c (6 srv)	3 c (6 srv)	3.5 c (7 srv)	3.5 c (7 srv)	4 c (8 srv)	4 c (8 srv)
Dark green veg.	3 c/wk	3 c/wk	3 c/wk	3 c/wk	3 c/wk	3 c/wk
Orange veg.	2 c/wk	2 c/wk	2.5 c/wk	2.5 c/wk	2.5 c/wk	2.5 c/wk
Legumes	3 c/wk	3 c/wk	3.5 c/wk	3.5 c/wk	3.5 c/wk	3.5 c/wk
Starchy veg.	6 c/wk	6 c/wk	7 c/wk	7 c/wk	9 c/wk	9 c/wk
Other veg.	7 c/wk	7 c/wk	8.5 c/wk	8.5 c/wk	10 c/wk	10 c/wk
Grains[4]	7 oz-eq	8 oz-eq	9 oz-eq	10 oz-eq	10 oz-eq	10 oz-eq
Whole grains	3.5	4	4.5	5	5	5
Other grains	3.5	4	4.5	5	5	5
Lean meat and beans	6 oz-eq	6.5 oz-eq	6.5 oz-eq	7 oz-eq	7 oz-eq	7 oz-eq
Milk	3 c	3 c	3 c	3 c	3 c	3 c
Oils[5]	29 g	31 g	34 g	36 g	44 g	51g
Discretionary calorie allowance[6]	290	362	410	426	512	648

Notes for Appendix A-2 continue on page 324

Notes for Appendix A-2:

[1] Food items included in each group and subgroup:

Fruits	All fresh, frozen, canned, and dried fruits and fruit juices: for example, oranges and orange juice, apples and apple juice, bananas, grapes, melons, berries, raisins. In developing the food patterns, only fruits and juices with no added sugars or fats were used. *See note 6 on discretionary calories if products with added sugars or fats are consumed.*
Vegetables	In developing the food patterns, only vegetables with no added fats or sugars were used. *See note 6 on discretionary calories if products with added fats or sugars are consumed.*
• Dark green vegetables	All fresh, frozen, and canned dark green vegetables, cooked or raw: for example, broccoli; spinach; romaine; collard, turnip, and mustard greens.
• Orange vegetables	All fresh, frozen, and canned orange and deep yellow vegetables, cooked or raw: for example, carrots, sweetpotatoes, winter squash, and pumpkin.
• Legumes (dry beans and peas)	All cooked dry beans and peas and soybean products: for example, pinto beans, kidney beans, lentils, chickpeas, tofu. (See comment under meat and beans group about counting legumes in the vegetable or the meat and beans group.)
• Starchy vegetables	All fresh, frozen, and canned starchy vegetables: for example, white potatoes, corn, green peas.
• Other vegetables	All fresh, frozen, and canned other vegetables, cooked or raw: for example, tomatoes, tomato juice, lettuce, green beans, onions.
Grains	In developing the food patterns, only grains in low-fat and low-sugar forms were used. *See note 6 on discretionary calories if products that are higher in fat and/or added sugars are consumed.*
• Whole grains	All whole-grain products and whole grains used as ingredients: for example, whole-wheat and rye breads, whole-grain cereals and crackers, oatmeal, and brown rice.
• Other grains	All refined grain products and refined grains used as ingredients: for example, white breads, enriched grain cereals and crackers, enriched pasta, white rice.
Meat, poultry, fish, dry beans, eggs, and nuts (meat & beans)	All meat, poultry, fish, dry beans and peas, eggs, nuts, seeds. Most choices should be lean or low-fat. *See note 6 on discretionary calories if higher fat products are consumed.* Dry beans and peas and soybean products are considered part of this group as well as the vegetable group, but should be counted in one group only.
Milk, yogurt, and cheese (milk)	All milks, yogurts, frozen yogurts, dairy desserts, cheeses (except cream cheese), including lactose-free and lactose-reduced products. Most choices should be fat-free or low-fat. In developing the food patterns, only fat-free milk was used. *See note 6 on discretionary calories if low-fat, reduced-fat, or whole milk or milk products—or milk products that contain added sugars—are consumed.* Calcium-fortified soy beverages are an option for those who want a non-dairy calcium source.

[2] Quantity equivalents for each food group:

Grains	The following each count as 1 ounce-equivalent (1 serving) of grains: $1/2$ cup cooked rice, pasta, or cooked cereal; 1 ounce dry pasta or rice; 1 slice bread; 1 small muffin (1 oz); 1 cup ready-to-eat cereal flakes.
Fruits and vegetables	The following each count as 1 cup (2 servings) of fruits or vegetables: 1 cup cut-up raw or cooked fruit or vegetable, 1 cup fruit or vegetable juice, 2 cups leafy salad greens.
Meat and beans	The following each count as 1 ounce-equivalent: 1 ounce lean meat, poultry, or fish; 1 egg; $1/4$ cup cooked dry beans or tofu; 1 Tbsp peanut butter; $1/2$ ounce nuts or seeds.
Milk	The following each count as 1 cup (1 serving) of milk: 1 cup milk or yogurt, $1\,1/2$ ounces natural cheese such as Cheddar cheese or 2 ounces processed cheese. Discretionary calories must be counted for all choices, except fat-free milk.

[3] Explanation of vegetable subgroup amounts: Vegetable subgroup amounts are shown in this table as weekly amounts, because it would be difficult for consumers to select foods from each subgroup daily. A daily amount that is one-seventh of the weekly amount listed is used in calculations of nutrient and energy levels in each pattern.

[4] Explanation of grain subgroup amounts: The whole grain subgroup amounts shown in this table represent at least three 1-ounce servings and one-half of the total amount as whole grains for all calorie levels of 1,600 and above. This is the minimum suggested amount of whole grains to consume as part of the food patterns. More whole grains up to all of the grains recommended may be selected, with offsetting decreases in the amounts of other (enriched) grains. In patterns designed for younger children (1,000, 1,200, and 1,400 calories), one-half of the total amount of grains is shown as whole grains.

Notes for Appendix A-2 continue on page 325

Notes for Appendix A-2: Continued

5 Explanation of oils: Oils (including soft margarine with zero *trans* fat) shown in this table represent the amounts that are added to foods during processing, cooking, or at the table. Oils and soft margarines include vegetable oils and soft vegetable oil table spreads that have no *trans* fats. The amounts of oils listed in this table are not considered to be part of discretionary calories because they are a major source of the vitamin E and polyunsaturated fatty acids, including the essential fatty acids, in the food pattern. In contrast, solid fats are listed separately in the discretionary calorie table (appendix A-3) because, compared with oils, they are higher in saturated fatty acids and lower in vitamin E and polyunsaturated and monounsaturated fatty acids, including essential fatty acids. The amounts of each type of fat in the food intake pattern were based on 60% oils and/or soft margarines with no *trans* fats and 40% solid fat. The amounts in typical American diets are about 42% oils or soft margarines and about 58% solid fats.

6 Explanation of discretionary calorie allowance: The discretionary calorie allowance is the remaining amount of calories in each food pattern after selecting the specified number of nutrient-dense forms of foods in each food group. The number of discretionary calories assumes that food items in each food group are selected in nutrient-dense forms (that is, forms that are fat-free or low-fat and that contain no added sugars). Solid fat and sugar calories always need to be counted as discretionary calories, as in the following examples:

• The fat in low-fat, reduced fat, or whole milk or milk products or cheese and the sugar and fat in chocolate milk, ice cream, pudding, etc.
• The fat in higher fat meats (e.g., ground beef with more than 5% fat by weight, poultry with skin, higher fat luncheon meats, sausages)
• The sugars added to fruits and fruit juices with added sugars or fruits canned in syrup
• The added fat and/or sugars in vegetables prepared with added fat or sugars
• The added fats and/or sugars in grain products containing higher levels of fats and/or sugars (e.g., sweetened cereals, higher fat crackers, pies and other pastries, cakes, cookies)

Total discretionary calories should be limited to the amounts shown in the table at each calorie level. The number of discretionary calories is lower in the 1,600-calorie pattern than in the 1,000-, 1,200-, and 1,400-calorie patterns. These lower calorie patterns are designed to meet the nutrient needs of children 2 to 8 years old. The nutrient goals for the 1,600-calorie pattern are set to meet the needs of adult women, which are higher and require that more calories be used in selections from the basic food groups. Additional information about discretionary calories, including an example of the division of these calories between solid fats and added sugars, is provided in appendix A-3.

Appendix A-3. Discretionary Calorie Allowance in the USDA Food Guide

The discretionary calorie allowance is the remaining amount of calories in each calorie level after nutrient-dense forms of foods in each food group are selected. This table shows the number of discretionary calories remaining in each calorie level if nutrient-dense foods are selected. Those trying to lose weight may choose not to use discretionary calories. For those wanting to maintain their weight, discretionary calories may be used to increase the amount of food selected from each food group; to consume foods that are not in the lowest fat form (such as 2% milk or medium-fat meat) or that contain added sugars; to add oil, fat, or sugars to foods; or to consume alcohol. The table shows an example of how these calories may be divided between solid fats and added sugars.

Discretionary calories that remain at each calorie level												
Food Guide calorie level	1,000	1,200	1,400	1,600	1,800	2,000	2,200	2,400	2,600	2,800	3,000	3,200
Discretionary calories[1]	165	171	171	132	195	267	290	362	410	426	512	648
Example of division of discretionary calories: Solid fats are shown in grams (g); added sugars in grams (g) and teaspoons (tsp).												
Solid fats[2]	11 g	14 g	14 g	11 g	15 g	18 g	19 g	22 g	24 g	24 g	29 g	34 g
Added sugars[3]	20 g (5 tsp)	16 g (4 tsp)	16 g (4 tsp)	12 g (3 tsp)	20 g (5 tsp)	32 g (8 tsp)	36 g (9 tsp)	48 g (12 tsp)	56 g (14 tsp)	60 g (15 tsp)	72g (18 tsp)	96 g (24 tsp)

[1] Discretionary calories: In developing the Food Guide, food items in nutrient-dense forms (that is, forms that are fat-free or low-fat and that contain no added sugars) were used. The number of discretionary calories assumes that food items in each food group are selected in nutrient-dense forms. Solid fat and sugar calories always need to be counted as discretionary calories, as in the following examples:
  • The fat in low-fat, reduced fat, or whole milk or milk products or cheese and the sugar and fat in chocolate milk, ice cream, pudding, etc.
  • The fat in higher fat meats (e.g., ground beef with more than 5% fat by weight, poultry with skin, higher fat luncheon meats, sausages)
  • The sugars added to fruits and fruit juices with added sugars or fruits canned in syrup
  • The added fat and/or sugars in vegetables prepared with added fat or sugars
  • The added fats and/or sugars in grain products containing higher levels of fats and/or sugars (e.g., sweetened cereals, higher fat crackers, pies and other pastries, cakes, cookies)

Total discretionary calories should be limited to the amounts shown in the table at each calorie level. The number of discretionary calories is lower in the 1,600-calorie pattern than in the 1,000, 1,200, and 1,400-calorie patterns. These lower calorie patterns are designed to meet the nutrient needs of children 2 to 8 years old. The nutrient goals for the 1,600-calorie pattern are set to meet the needs of adult women, which are higher and require that more calories be used in selections from the basic food groups. The calories assigned to discretionary calories may be used to increase intake from the basic food groups; to select foods from these groups that are higher in fat or with added sugars; to add oils, solid fats, or sugars to foods or beverages; or to consume alcohol. See note 2 on limits for solid fats.

[2] Solid fats: Amounts of solid fats listed in the table represent about 7 to 8% of calories from saturated fat. Foods in each food group are represented in their lowest fat forms, such as fat-free milk and skinless chicken. Solid fats shown in this table represent the amounts of fats that may be added in cooking or at the table, and fats consumed when higher fat items are selected from the food groups (e.g., whole milk instead of fat-free milk, chicken with skin, or cookies instead of bread), without exceeding the recommended

Notes for Appendix A-3 continue on page 327

Notes for Appendix A-3: Continued

limits on saturated fat intake. Solid fats include meat and poultry fats eaten either as part of the meat or poultry product or separately; milk fat such as that in whole milk, cheese, and butter; shortenings used in baked products; and hard margarines.

Solid fats and oils are separated because their fatty acid compositions differ. Solid fats are higher in saturated fatty acids, and commonly consumed oils and soft margarines with no *trans* fats are higher in vitamin E and polyunsaturated and monounsaturated fatty acids, including essential fatty acids. Oils listed in appendix A-2 are not considered to be part of the discretionary calorie allowance because they are a major source of the essential fatty acids and vitamin E in the food pattern.

The gram weights for solid fats are the amounts of these products that can be included in the pattern and are not identical to the amount of lipids in these items, because some products (margarines, butter) contain water or other ingredients, in addition to lipids.

[3] Added sugars: Added sugars are the sugars and syrups added to foods and beverages in processing or preparation, not the naturally occurring sugars in fruits or milk. The amounts of added sugars suggested in the example are NOT specific recommendations for amounts of added sugars to consume, but rather represent the amounts that can be included at each calorie level without over-consuming calories. The suggested amounts of added sugars may be helpful as part of the Food Guide to allow for some sweetened foods or beverages, without exceeding energy needs. This use of added sugars as a calorie balance requires two assumptions: (1) that selections are made from all food groups in accordance with the suggested amounts and (2) that additional fats are used in the amounts shown, which, together with the fats in the core food groups, represent about 27-30% of calories from fat.

APPENDIX B. FOOD SOURCES OF SELECTED NUTRIENTS

Appendix B-1. Food Sources of Potassium

Food Sources of Potassium ranked by milligrams of potassium per standard amount, also showing calories in the standard amount. (The AI for adults is 4,700 mg/day potassium.)

Food, Standard Amount	Potassium (mg)	Calories
Sweetpotato, baked, 1 potato (146 g)	694	131
Tomato paste, 1/4 cup	664	54
Beet greens, cooked, 1/2 cup	655	19
Potato, baked, flesh, 1 potato (156 g)	610	145
White beans, canned, 1/2 cup	595	153
Yogurt, plain, non-fat, 8-oz container	579	127
Tomato puree, 1/2 cup	549	48
Clams, canned, 3 oz	534	126
Yogurt, plain, low-fat, 8-oz container	531	143
Prune juice, 3/4 cup	530	136
Carrot juice, 3/4 cup	517	71
Blackstrap molasses, 1 Tbsp	498	47
Halibut, cooked, 3 oz	490	119
Soybeans, green, cooked, 1/2 cup	485	127
Tuna, yellowfin, cooked, 3 oz	484	118
Lima beans, cooked, 1/2 cup	484	104
Winter squash, cooked, 1/2 cup	448	40
Soybeans, mature, cooked, 1/2 cup	443	149
Rockfish, Pacific, cooked, 3 oz	442	103
Cod, Pacific, cooked, 3 oz	439	89
Bananas, 1 medium	422	105
Spinach, cooked, 1/2 cup	419	21
Tomato juice, 3/4 cup	417	31
Tomato sauce, 1/2 cup	405	39
Peaches, dried, uncooked, 1/4 cup	398	96
Prunes, stewed, 1/2 cup	398	133
Milk, non-fat, 1 cup	382	83

Appendix B-1 continues on page 329

Appendix B-1: Continued

Food, Standard Amount	Potassium (mg)	Calories
Pork chop, center loin, cooked, 3 oz	382	197
Apricots, dried, uncooked, 1/4 cup	378	78
Rainbow trout, farmed, cooked, 3 oz	375	144
Pork loin, center rib (roasts), lean, roasted, 3 oz	371	190
Buttermilk, cultured, low-fat, 1 cup	370	98
Cantaloupe, 1/4 medium	368	47
1%–2% milk, 1 cup	366	102–122
Honeydew melon, 1/8 medium	365	58
Lentils, cooked, 1/2 cup	365	115
Plantains, cooked, 1/2 cup slices	358	90
Kidney beans, cooked, 1/2 cup	358	112
Orange juice, 3/4 cup	355	85
Split peas, cooked, 1/2 cup	355	116
Yogurt, plain, whole milk, 8 oz container	352	138

Source: Nutrient values from Agricultural Research Service (ARS) Nutrient Database for Standard Reference, Release 17. Foods are from ARS single nutrient reports, sorted in descending order by nutrient content in terms of common household measures. Food items and weights in the single nutrient reports are adapted from those in 2002 revision of USDA Home and Garden Bulletin No. 72, Nutritive Value of Foods. Mixed dishes and multiple preparations of the same food item have been omitted from this table.

Appendix B-2. Food Sources of Vitamin E

Food Sources of Vitamin E ranked by milligrams of vitamin E per standard amount; also calories in the standard amount. (All provide ≥ 10% of RDA for vitamin E for adults, which is 15 mg α–tocopherol [AT]/day.)

Food, Standard Amount	AT (mg)	Calories
Fortified ready-to-eat cereals, ~ 1 oz	1.6–12.8	90–107
Sunflower seeds, dry roasted, 1 oz	7.4	165
Almonds, 1 oz	7.3	164
Sunflower oil, high linoleic, 1 Tbsp	5.6	120
Cottonseed oil, 1 Tbsp	4.8	120
Safflower oil, high oleic, 1 Tbsp	4.6	120
Hazelnuts (filberts), 1 oz	4.3	178
Mixed nuts, dry roasted, 1 oz	3.1	168
Turnip greens, frozen, cooked, 1/2 cup	2.9	24
Tomato paste, 1/4 cup	2.8	54
Pine nuts, 1 oz	2.6	191
Peanut butter, 2 Tbsp	2.5	192
Tomato puree, 1/2 cup	2.5	48
Tomato sauce, 1/2 cup	2.5	39
Canola oil, 1 Tbsp	2.4	124
Wheat germ, toasted, plain, 2 Tbsp	2.3	54
Peanuts, 1 oz	2.2	166
Avocado, raw, 1/2 avocado	2.1	161
Carrot juice, canned, 3/4 cup	2.1	71
Peanut oil, 1 Tbsp	2.1	119
Corn oil, 1 Tbsp	1.9	120
Olive oil, 1 Tbsp	1.9	119
Spinach, cooked, 1/2 cup	1.9	21
Dandelion greens, cooked, 1/2 cup	1.8	18
Sardine, Atlantic, in oil, drained, 3 oz	1.7	177
Blue crab, cooked/canned, 3 oz	1.6	84
Brazil nuts, 1 oz	1.6	186
Herring, Atlantic, pickled, 3 oz	1.5	222

Source: Nutrient values from Agricultural Research Service (ARS) Nutrient Database for Standard Reference, Release 17. Foods are from ARS single nutrient reports, sorted in descending order by nutrient content in terms of common household measures. Food items and weights in the single nutrient reports are adapted from those in 2002 revision of USDA Home and Garden Bulletin No. 72, Nutritive Value of Foods. Mixed dishes and multiple preparations of the same food item have been omitted from this table.

Appendix B-3. Food Sources of Iron

Food Sources of Iron ranked by milligrams of iron per standard amount; also calories in the standard amount. (All are ≥ 10% of RDA for teen and adult females, which is 18 mg/day.)

Food, Standard Amount	Iron (mg)	Calories
Clams, canned, drained, 3 oz	23.8	126
Fortified ready-to-eat cereals (various), ~ 1 oz	1.8 –21.1	54–127
Oysters, eastern, wild, cooked, moist heat, 3 oz	10.2	116
Organ meats (liver, giblets), various, cooked, 3 oz [a]	5.2–9.9	134–235
Fortified instant cooked cereals (various), 1 packet	4.9–8.1	Varies
Soybeans, mature, cooked, 1/2 cup	4.4	149
Pumpkin and squash seed kernels, roasted, 1 oz	4.2	148
White beans, canned, 1/2 cup	3.9	153
Blackstrap molasses, 1 Tbsp	3.5	47
Lentils, cooked, 1/2 cup	3.3	115
Spinach, cooked from fresh, 1/2 cup	3.2	21
Beef, chuck, blade roast, lean, cooked, 3 oz	3.1	215
Beef, bottom round, lean, 0" fat, all grades, cooked, 3 oz	2.8	182
Kidney beans, cooked, 1/2 cup	2.6	112
Sardines, canned in oil, drained, 3 oz	2.5	177
Beef, rib, lean, 1/4" fat, all grades, 3 oz	2.4	195
Chickpeas, cooked, 1/2 cup	2.4	134
Duck, meat only, roasted, 3 oz	2.3	171
Lamb, shoulder, arm, lean, 1/4" fat, choice, cooked, 3 oz	2.3	237
Prune juice, 3/4 cup	2.3	136
Shrimp, canned, 3 oz	2.3	102
Cowpeas, cooked, 1/2 cup	2.2	100
Ground beef, 15% fat, cooked, 3 oz	2.2	212
Tomato puree, 1/2 cup	2.2	48
Lima beans, cooked, 1/2 cup	2.2	108
Soybeans, green, cooked, 1/2 cup	2.2	127
Navy beans, cooked, 1/2 cup	2.1	127
Refried beans, 1/2 cup	2.1	118
Beef, top sirloin, lean, 0" fat, all grades, cooked, 3 oz	2.0	156
Tomato paste, 1/4 cup	2.0	54

[a] High in cholesterol.

Source: Nutrient values from Agricultural Research Service (ARS) Nutrient Database for Standard Reference, Release 17. Foods are from ARS single nutrient reports, sorted in descending order by nutrient content in terms of common household measures. Food items and weights in the single nutrient reports are adapted from those in 2002 revision of USDA Home and Garden Bulletin No. 72, Nutritive Value of Foods. Mixed dishes and multiple preparations of the same food item have been omitted from this table.

Appendix B-4. Non-Dairy Food Sources of Calcium

Non-Dairy Food Sources of Calcium ranked by milligrams of calcium per standard amount; also calories in the standard amount. The bioavailability may vary. (The AI for adults is 1,000 mg/day.)[a]

Food, Standard Amount	Calcium (mg)	Calories
Fortified ready-to-eat cereals (various), 1 oz	236–1043	88–106
Soy beverage, calcium fortified, 1 cup	368	98
Sardines, Atlantic, in oil, drained, 3 oz	325	177
Tofu, firm, prepared with nigari[b], 1/2 cup	253	88
Pink salmon, canned, with bone, 3 oz	181	118
Collards, cooked from frozen, 1/2 cup	178	31
Molasses, blackstrap, 1 Tbsp	172	47
Spinach, cooked from frozen, 1/2 cup	146	30
Soybeans, green, cooked, 1/2 cup	130	127
Turnip greens, cooked from frozen, 1/2 cup	124	24
Ocean perch, Atlantic, cooked, 3 oz	116	103
Oatmeal, plain and flavored, instant, fortified, 1 packet prepared	99–110	97–157
Cowpeas, cooked, 1/2 cup	106	80
White beans, canned, 1/2 cup	96	153
Kale, cooked from frozen, 1/2 cup	90	20
Okra, cooked from frozen, 1/2 cup	88	26
Soybeans, mature, cooked, 1/2 cup	88	149
Blue crab, canned, 3 oz	86	84
Beet greens, cooked from fresh, 1/2 cup	82	19
Pak-choi, Chinese cabbage, cooked from fresh, 1/2 cup	79	10
Clams, canned, 3 oz	78	126
Dandelion greens, cooked from fresh, 1/2 cup	74	17
Rainbow trout, farmed, cooked, 3 oz	73	144

[a] Both calcium content and bioavailability should be considered when selecting dietary sources of calcium. Some plant foods have calcium that is well absorbed, but the large quantity of plant foods that would be needed to provide as much calcium as in a glass of milk may be unachievable for many. Many other calcium-fortified foods are available, but the percentage of calcium that can be absorbed is unavailable for many of them.

[b] Calcium sulfate and magnesium chloride.

Source: Nutrient values from Agricultural Research Service (ARS) Nutrient Database for Standard Reference, Release 17. Foods are from ARS single nutrient reports, sorted in descending order by nutrient content in terms of common household measures. Food items and weights in the single nutrient reports are adapted from those in 2002 revision of USDA Home and Garden Bulletin No. 72, Nutritive Value of Foods. Mixed dishes and multiple preparations of the same food item have been omitted from this table.

Appendix B-5. Food Sources of Calcium

Food Sources of Calcium ranked by milligrams of calcium per standard amount; also calories in the standard amount. (All are ≥20% of AI for adults 19-50, which is 1,000 mg/day.)

Food, Standard Amount	Calcium (mg)	Calories
Plain yogurt, non-fat (13 g protein/8 oz), 8-oz container	452	127
Romano cheese, 1.5 oz	452	165
Pasteurized process Swiss cheese, 2 oz	438	190
Plain yogurt, low-fat (12 g protein/8 oz), 8-oz container	415	143
Fruit yogurt, low-fat (10 g protein/8 oz), 8-oz container	345	232
Swiss cheese, 1.5 oz	336	162
Ricotta cheese, part skim, 1/2 cup	335	170
Pasteurized process American cheese food, 2 oz	323	188
Provolone cheese, 1.5 oz	321	150
Mozzarella cheese, part-skim, 1.5 oz	311	129
Cheddar cheese, 1.5 oz	307	171
Fat-free (skim) milk, 1 cup	306	83
Muenster cheese, 1.5 oz	305	156
1% low-fat milk, 1 cup	290	102
Low-fat chocolate milk (1%), 1 cup	288	158
2% reduced fat milk, 1 cup	285	122
Reduced fat chocolate milk (2%), 1 cup	285	180
Buttermilk, low-fat, 1 cup	284	98
Chocolate milk, 1 cup	280	208
Whole milk, 1 cup	276	146
Yogurt, plain, whole milk (8 g protein/8 oz), 8-oz container	275	138
Ricotta cheese, whole milk, 1/2 cup	255	214
Blue cheese, 1.5 oz	225	150
Mozzarella cheese, whole milk, 1.5 oz	215	128
Feta cheese, 1.5 oz	210	113

Source: Nutrient values from Agricultural Research Service (ARS) Nutrient Database for Standard Reference, Release 17. Foods are from ARS single nutrient reports, sorted in descending order by nutrient content in terms of common household measures. Food items and weights in the single nutrient reports are adapted from those in 2002 revision of USDA Home and Garden Bulletin No. 72, Nutritive Value of Foods. Mixed dishes and multiple preparations of the same food item have been omitted from this table.

Appendix B-6. Food Sources of Vitamin A

Food Sources of Vitamin A ranked by micrograms Retinol Activity Equivalents (RAE) of vitamin A per standard amount; also calories in the standard amount. (All are ≥20% of RDA for adult men, which is 900 mg/day RAE.)

Food, Standard Amount	Vitamin A (μg RAE)	Calories
Organ meats (liver, giblets), various, cooked, 3 oz[a]	1490–9126	134–235
Carrot juice, 3/4 cup	1692	71
Sweetpotato with peel, baked, 1 medium	1096	103
Pumpkin, canned, 1/2 cup	953	42
Carrots, cooked from fresh, 1/2 cup	671	27
Spinach, cooked from frozen, 1/2 cup	573	30
Collards, cooked from frozen, 1/2 cup	489	31
Kale, cooked from frozen, 1/2 cup	478	20
Mixed vegetables, canned, 1/2 cup	474	40
Turnip greens, cooked from frozen, 1/2 cup	441	24
Instant cooked cereals, fortified, prepared, 1 packet	285–376	75–97
Various ready-to-eat cereals, with added vit. A, ~1 oz	180–376	100–117
Carrot, raw, 1 small	301	20
Beet greens, cooked, 1/2 cup	276	19
Winter squash, cooked, 1/2 cup	268	38
Dandelion greens, cooked, 1/2 cup	260	18
Cantaloupe, raw, 1/4 medium melon	233	46
Mustard greens, cooked, 1/2 cup	221	11
Pickled herring, 3 oz	219	222
Red sweet pepper, cooked, 1/2 cup	186	19
Chinese cabbage, cooked, 1/2 cup	180	10

[a] High in cholesterol.

Source: Nutrient values from Agricultural Research Service (ARS) Nutrient Database for Standard Reference, Release 17. Foods are from ARS single nutrient reports, sorted in descending order by nutrient content in terms of common household measures. Food items and weights in the single nutrient reports are adapted from those in 2002 revision of USDA Home and Garden Bulletin No. 72, Nutritive Value of Foods. Mixed dishes and multiple preparations of the same food item have been omitted from this table.

Appendix B-7. Food Sources of Magnesium

Food Sources of Magnesium ranked by milligrams of magnesium per standard amount; also calories in the standard amount. (All are ≥ 10% of RDA for adult men, which is 420 mg/day.)

Food, Standard Amount	Magnesium (mg)	Calories
Pumpkin and squash seed kernels, roasted, 1 oz	151	148
Brazil nuts, 1 oz	107	186
Bran ready-to-eat cereal (100%), ~1 oz	103	74
Halibut, cooked, 3 oz	91	119
Quinoa, dry, 1/4 cup	89	159
Spinach, canned, 1/2 cup	81	25
Almonds, 1 oz	78	164
Spinach, cooked from fresh, 1/2 cup	78	20
Buckwheat flour, 1/4 cup	75	101
Cashews, dry roasted, 1 oz	74	163
Soybeans, mature, cooked, 1/2 cup	74	149
Pine nuts, dried, 1 oz	71	191
Mixed nuts, oil roasted, with peanuts, 1 oz	67	175
White beans, canned, 1/2 cup	67	154
Pollock, walleye, cooked, 3 oz	62	96
Black beans, cooked, 1/2 cup	60	114
Bulgur, dry, 1/4 cup	57	120
Oat bran, raw, 1/4 cup	55	58
Soybeans, green, cooked, 1/2 cup	54	127
Tuna, yellowfin, cooked, 3 oz	54	118
Artichokes (hearts), cooked, 1/2 cup	50	42
Peanuts, dry roasted, 1 oz	50	166
Lima beans, baby, cooked from frozen, 1/2 cup	50	95
Beet greens, cooked, 1/2 cup	49	19
Navy beans, cooked, 1/2 cup	48	127
Tofu, firm, prepared with nigari[a], 1/2 cup	47	88
Okra, cooked from frozen, 1/2 cup	47	26
Soy beverage, 1 cup	47	127

Appendix B-7 continues on page 336

Appendix B-7: Continued

Food, Standard Amount	Magnesium (mg)	Calories
Cowpeas, cooked, 1/2 cup	46	100
Hazelnuts, 1 oz	46	178
Oat bran muffin, 1 oz	45	77
Great northern beans, cooked, 1/2 cup	44	104
Oat bran, cooked, 1/2 cup	44	44
Buckwheat groats, roasted, cooked, 1/2 cup	43	78
Brown rice, cooked, 1/2 cup	42	108
Haddock, cooked, 3 oz	42	95

a Calcium sulfate and magnesium chloride.

Source: Nutrient values from Agricultural Research Service (ARS) Nutrient Database for Standard Reference, Release 17. Foods are from ARS single nutrient reports, sorted in descending order by nutrient content in terms of common household measures. Food items and weights in the single nutrient reports are adapted from those in 2002 revision of USDA Home and Garden Bulletin No. 72, Nutritive Value of Foods. Mixed dishes and multiple preparations of the same food item have been omitted from this table.

Appendix B-8. Food Sources of Dietary Fiber

Food Sources of Dietary Fiber ranked by grams of dietary fiber per standard amount; also calories in the standard amount. (All are ≥10% of AI for adult women, which is 25 grams/day.)

Food, Standard Amount	Dietary Fiber (g)	Calories
Navy beans, cooked, 1/2 cup	9.5	128
Bran ready-to-eat cereal (100%), 1/2 cup	8.8	78
Kidney beans, canned, 1/2 cup	8.2	109
Split peas, cooked, 1/2 cup	8.1	116
Lentils, cooked, 1/2 cup	7.8	115
Black beans, cooked, 1/2 cup	7.5	114
Pinto beans, cooked, 1/2 cup	7.7	122
Lima beans, cooked, 1/2 cup	6.6	108
Artichoke, globe, cooked, 1 each	6.5	60
White beans, canned, 1/2 cup	6.3	154
Chickpeas, cooked, 1/2 cup	6.2	135
Great northern beans, cooked, 1/2 cup	6.2	105
Cowpeas, cooked, 1/2 cup	5.6	100
Soybeans, mature, cooked, 1/2 cup	5.2	149
Bran ready-to-eat cereals, various, ~1 oz	2.6–5.0	90–108
Crackers, rye wafers, plain, 2 wafers	5.0	74
Sweetpotato, baked, with peel, 1 medium (146 g)	4.8	131
Asian pear, raw, 1 small	4.4	51
Green peas, cooked, 1/2 cup	4.4	67
Whole-wheat English muffin, 1 each	4.4	134
Pear, raw, 1 small	4.3	81
Bulgur, cooked, 1/2 cup	4.1	76
Mixed vegetables, cooked, 1/2 cup	4.0	59
Raspberries, raw, 1/2 cup	4.0	32
Sweetpotato, boiled, no peel, 1 medium (156 g)	3.9	119
Blackberries, raw, 1/2 cup	3.8	31
Potato, baked, with skin, 1 medium	3.8	161
Soybeans, green, cooked, 1/2 cup	3.8	127
Stewed prunes, 1/2 cup	3.8	133
Figs, dried, 1/4 cup	3.7	93
Dates, 1/4 cup	3.6	126
Oat bran, raw, 1/4 cup	3.6	58

Appendix B-8 continues on page 338

Appendix B-8: Continued

Food, Standard Amount	Dietary Fiber (g)	Calories
Pumpkin, canned, 1/2 cup	3.6	42
Spinach, frozen, cooked, 1/2 cup	3.5	30
Shredded wheat ready-to-eat cereals, various, ~1 oz	2.8–3.4	96
Almonds, 1 oz	3.3	164
Apple with skin, raw, 1 medium	3.3	72
Brussels sprouts, frozen, cooked, 1/2 cup	3.2	33
Whole-wheat spaghetti, cooked, 1/2 cup	3.1	87
Banana, 1 medium	3.1	105
Orange, raw, 1 medium	3.1	62
Oat bran muffin, 1 small	3.0	178
Guava, 1 medium	3.0	37
Pearled barley, cooked, 1/2 cup	3.0	97
Sauerkraut, canned, solids, and liquids, 1/2 cup	3.0	23
Tomato paste, 1/4 cup	2.9	54
Winter squash, cooked, 1/2 cup	2.9	38
Broccoli, cooked, 1/2 cup	2.8	26
Parsnips, cooked, chopped, 1/2 cup	2.8	55
Turnip greens, cooked, 1/2 cup	2.5	15
Collards, cooked, 1/2 cup	2.7	25
Okra, frozen, cooked, 1/2 cup	2.6	26
Peas, edible-podded, cooked, 1/2 cup	2.5	42

Source: ARS Nutrient Database for Standard Reference, Release 17. Foods are from single nutrient reports, which are sorted either by food description or in descending order by nutrient content in terms of common household measures. The food items and weights in these reports are adapted from those in 2002 revision of USDA Home and Garden Bulletin No. 72, Nutritive Value of Foods. Mixed dishes and multiple preparations of the same food item have been omitted.

Appendix B-9. Food Sources of Vitamin C

Food Sources of Vitamin C ranked by milligrams of vitamin C per standard amount; also calories in the standard amount. (All provide ≥20% of RDA for adult men, which is 90 mg/day.)

Food, Standard Amount	Vitamin C (mg)	Calories
Guava, raw, 1/2 cup	188	56
Red sweet pepper, raw, 1/2 cup	142	20
Red sweet pepper, cooked, 1/2 cup	116	19
Kiwi fruit, 1 medium	70	46
Orange, raw, 1 medium	70	62
Orange juice, 3/4 cup	61–93	79–84
Green pepper, sweet, raw, 1/2 cup	60	15
Green pepper, sweet, cooked, 1/2 cup	51	19
Grapefruit juice, 3/4 cup	50–70	71–86
Vegetable juice cocktail, 3/4 cup	50	34
Strawberries, raw, 1/2 cup	49	27
Brussels sprouts, cooked, 1/2 cup	48	28
Cantaloupe, 1/4 medium	47	51
Papaya, raw, 1/4 medium	47	30
Kohlrabi, cooked, 1/2 cup	45	24
Broccoli, raw, 1/2 cup	39	15
Edible pod peas, cooked, 1/2 cup	38	34
Broccoli, cooked, 1/2 cup	37	26
Sweetpotato, canned, 1/2 cup	34	116
Tomato juice, 3/4 cup	33	31
Cauliflower, cooked, 1/2 cup	28	17
Pineapple, raw, 1/2 cup	28	37
Kale, cooked, 1/2 cup	27	18
Mango, 1/2 cup	23	54

Source: Nutrient values from Agricultural Research Service (ARS) Nutrient Database for Standard Reference, Release 17. Foods are from ARS single nutrient reports, sorted in descending order by nutrient content in terms of common household measures. Food items and weights in the single nutrient reports are adapted from those in 2002 revision of USDA Home and Garden Bulletin No. 72, Nutritive Value of Foods. Mixed dishes and multiple preparations of the same food item have been omitted from this table.

APPENDIX C. GLOSSARY OF TERMS

Acceptable Macronutrient Distribution Ranges (AMDR)—Range of intake for a particular energy source that is associated with reduced risk of chronic disease while providing intakes of essential nutrients. If an individual consumes in excess of the AMDR, there is a potential of increasing the risk of chronic diseases and/or insufficient intakes of essential nutrients.

Added Sugars—Sugars and syrups that are added to foods during processing or preparation. Added sugars do not include naturally occurring sugars such as those that occur in milk and fruits.

Adequate Intakes (AI)—A recommended average daily nutrient intake level based on observed or experimentally determined approximations or estimates of mean nutrient intake by a group (or groups) of apparently healthy people. The AI is used when the Estimated Average Requirement cannot be determined.

Basic Food Groups—In the USDA food intake patterns, the basic food groups are grains; fruits; vegetables; milk, yogurt, and cheese; and meat, poultry, fish, dried peas and beans, eggs, and nuts. In the DASH Eating Plan, nuts, seeds, and dry beans are a separate food group from meat, poultry, fish, and eggs.

Body Mass Index (BMI)—BMI is a practical measure for approximating total body fat and is a measure of weight in relation to height. It is calculated as weight in kilograms divided by the square of the height in meters.

Cardiovascular Disease—Refers to diseases of the heart and diseases of the blood vessel system (arteries, capillaries, veins) within a person's entire body, such as the brain, legs, and lungs.

Cholesterol—A sterol present in all animal tissues. Free cholesterol is a component of cell membranes and serves as a precursor for steroid hormones, including estrogen, testosterone, aldosterone, and bile acids. Humans are able to synthesize sufficient cholesterol to meet biologic requirements, and there is no evidence for a dietary requirement for cholesterol.

- **Dietary cholesterol**—Consumed from foods of animal origin, including meat, fish, poultry, eggs, and dairy products. Plant foods, such as grains, fruits and vegetables, and oils from these sources contain no dietary cholesterol.
- **Serum cholesterol**—Travels in the blood in distinct particles containing both lipids and proteins. Three major classes of lipoproteins are found in the serum of a fasting individual: low-density lipoprotein (LDL), high-density lipoprotein (HDL), and very-low-density lipoprotein (VLDL). Another lipoprotein class, intermediate-density lipoprotein (IDL), resides between VLDL and LDL; in clinical practice, IDL is included in the LDL measurement.

Chronic Diseases—such as heart disease, cancer, and diabetes—are the leading causes of death and disability in the United States. These diseases account for 7 of every 10 deaths and affect the quality of life of 90 million Americans. Although chronic diseases are among the most common and costly health problems, they are also among the most preventable. Adopting healthy behaviors such as eating nutritious foods, being physically active, and avoiding tobacco use can prevent or control the devastating effects of these diseases.

Coronary Heart Disease—A narrowing of the small blood vessels that supply blood and oxygen to the heart (coronary arteries).

Daily Food Intake Pattern—Identifies the types and amounts of foods that are recommended to be eaten each day and that meet specific nutritional goals. (*Federal Register Notice*, vol. 68, no. 176, p. 53536, Thursday, September 11, 2003)

Danger Zone—The temperature that allows bacteria to multiply rapidly and produce toxins, between 40°F and 140°F. To keep food out of this danger zone, keep cold food cold and hot food hot. Keep food cold in the refrigerator, in coolers, or on ice in the service line. Keep hot food in the oven, in heated chafing dishes, or in preheated steam tables, warming trays, and/or slow cookers. Never leave perishable foods, such as meat, poultry, eggs, and casseroles, in the danger zone longer than 2 hours or longer than 1 hour in temperatures above 90°F.

Dietary Fiber—Nonstarch polysaccharides and lignin that are not digested by enzymes in the small intestine. Dietary fiber typically refers to nondigestible carbohydrates from plant foods.

Dietary Reference Intakes (DRIs)—A set of nutrient-based reference values that expand upon and replace the former Recommended Dietary Allowances (RDAs) in the United States and the Recommended Nutrient Intakes (RNIs) in Canada. They are actually a set of four reference values: Estimated Average Requirements (EARs), RDAs, AIs, and Tolerable Upper Intake Levels (ULs).

Discretionary Calorie Allowance—The balance of calories remaining in a person's energy allowance after accounting for the number of calories needed to meet recommended nutrient intakes through consumption of foods in low-fat or no-added-sugar forms. The discretionary calorie allowance may be used in selecting forms of foods that are not the most nutrient-dense (e.g., whole milk rather than fat-free milk) or may be additions to foods (e.g., salad dressing, sugar, butter).

Energy Allowance—A person's energy allowance is the calorie intake at which weight maintenance occurs.

Estimated Average Requirements—EAR is the average daily nutrient intake level estimated to meet the requirement of half the healthy individuals in a particular life stage and gender group.

Estimated Energy Requirement—The EER represents the average dietary energy intake that will maintain energy balance in a healthy person of a given gender, age, weight, height, and physical activity level.

FDAMA—The Food and Drug Administration Modernization Act, enacted Nov. 21, 1997, amended the Federal Food, Drug, and Cosmetic Act relating to the regulation of food, drugs, devices, and biological products. With the passage of FDAMA, Congress enhanced FDA's mission in ways that recognized the Agency would be operating in a 21st century characterized by increasing technological, trade, and public health complexities.

FightBAC!—A national public education campaign to promote food safety to consumers and educate them on how to handle and prepare food safely. In this campaign, pathogens are represented by a cartoon-like bacteria character named "BAC."

Foodborne Disease—Caused by consuming contaminated foods or beverages. Many different disease-causing microbes, or pathogens, can contaminate foods, so there are many different foodborne infections. In addition, poisonous chemicals, or other harmful substances, can cause foodborne diseases if they are present in food. The most commonly recognized foodborne infections are those caused by the bacteria *Campylobacter, Salmonella,* and *E. coli* O157:H7, and by a group of viruses called calicivirus, also known as the Norwalk and Norwalk-like viruses.

Heme Iron—One of two forms of iron occurring in foods. Heme iron is bound within the iron-carrying proteins (hemoglobin and myoglobin) found in meat, poultry, and fish. While it contributes a smaller portion of iron to typical American diets than non-heme iron, a larger proportion of heme iron is absorbed

High-Fructose Corn Syrup (HFCS)—A corn sweetener derived from the wet milling of corn. Cornstarch is converted to a syrup that is nearly all dextrose. HFCS is found in numerous foods and beverages on the grocery store shelves.

Hydrogenation—A chemical reaction that adds hydrogen atoms to an unsaturated fat, thus saturating it and making it solid at room temperature.

Leisure-Time Physical Activity—Physical activity that is performed during exercise, recreation, or any additional time other than that associated with one's regular job duties, occupation, or transportation.

Listeriosis—A serious infection caused by eating food contaminated with the bacterium *Listeria monocytogenes*, which has recently been recognized as an important public health problem in the United States. The disease affects primarily pregnant women, their fetuses, newborns, and adults with weakened immune systems. Listeria is killed by pasteurization and cooking; however, in certain ready-to-eat foods, such as hot dogs and deli meats, contamination may occur after cooking/manufacture but before packaging. *Listeria monocytogenes* can survive at refrigerated temperatures.

Macronutrient—The dietary macronutrient groups are carbohydrates, proteins, and fats.

Micronutrient—Vitamins and minerals that are required in the human diet in very small amounts.

Moderate Physical Activity—Any activity that burns 3.5 to 7 kcal/min or the equivalent of 3 to 6 metabolic equivalents (METs) and results in achieving 60 to 73 percent of peak heart rate. An estimate of a person's peak heart rate can be obtained by subtracting the person's age from 220. Examples of moderate physical activity include walking briskly, mowing the lawn, dancing, swimming, or bicycling on level terrain. A person should feel some exertion but should be able to carry on a conversation comfortably during the activity.

Monounsaturated Fatty Acids—Monounsaturated fatty acids (MUFAs) have one double bond. Plant sources that are rich in MUFAs include vegetable oils (e.g., canola oil, olive oil, high oleic safflower and sunflower oils) that are liquid at room temperature and nuts.

Nutrient-Dense Foods—Nutrient-dense foods are those that provide substantial amounts of vitamins and minerals and relatively fewer calories.

Ounce-Equivalent—In the grains food group, the amount of a food counted as equal to a one-ounce slice of bread; in the meat, poultry, fish, dry beans, eggs, and nuts food group, the amount of food counted as equal to one ounce of cooked meat, poultry, or fish. Examples are listed in table 1 and appendix A-1.

n-6 PUFAs—Linoleic acid, one of the n-6 fatty acids, is required but cannot be synthesized by humans and, therefore, is considered essential in the diet. Primary sources are liquid vegetable oils, including soybean oil, corn oil, and safflower oil.

n-3 PUFAs—α-linolenic acid is an n-3 fatty acid that is required because it is not synthesized by humans and, therefore, is considered essential in the diet. It is obtained from plant sources, including soybean oil, canola oil, walnuts, and flaxseed. Eicosapentaenoic acid (EPA) and docosahexaenoic acid (DHA) are long-chain n-3 fatty acids that are contained in fish and shellfish.

Pathogen—Any microorganism that can cause or is capable of causing disease.

Polyunsaturated Fatty Acids—Polyunsaturated fatty acids (PUFAs) have two or more double bonds and may be of two types, based on the position of the first double bond.

Portion Size—The amount of a food consumed in one eating occasion.

Recommended Dietary Allowance (RDA)—The dietary intake level that is sufficient to meet the nutrient requirement of nearly all (97 to 98 percent) healthy individuals in a particular life stage and gender group.

Resistance Exercise—Anaerobic training, including weight training, weight machine use, and resistance band workouts. Resistance training will increase strength, muscular endurance, and muscle size, while running and jogging will not.

Saturated Fatty Acids—Saturated fatty acids have no double bonds. They primarily come from animal products such as meat and dairy products. In general, animal fats are solid at room temperature.

Sedentary Behaviors—In scientific literature, sedentary is often defined in terms of little or no physical activity during leisure time. A sedentary lifestyle is a lifestyle characterized by little or no physical activity.

Serving Size—A standardized amount of a food, such as a cup or an ounce, used in providing dietary guidance or in making comparisons among similar foods.

Tolerable Upper Intake Level (UL)—The highest average daily nutrient intake level likely to pose no risk of adverse health effects for nearly all individuals in a particular life stage and gender group. As intake increases above the UL, the potential risk of adverse health effects increases.

Trans **fatty acids**—*Trans* fatty acids, or *trans* fats, are unsaturated fatty acids that contain at least one non-conjugated double bond in the *trans* configuration. Sources of *trans* fatty acids include hydrogenated/partially hydrogenated vegetable oils that are used to make shortening and commercially prepared baked goods, snack foods, fried foods, and margarine. *Trans* fatty acids also are present in foods that come from ruminant animals (e.g., cattle and sheep). Such foods include dairy products, beef, and lamb.

Vegetarian—There are several categories of vegetarians, all of whom avoid meat and/or animal products. The vegan or total vegetarian diet includes only foods from plants: fruits, vegetables, legumes (dried beans and peas), grains, seeds, and nuts. The lactovegetarian diet includes plant foods plus cheese and other dairy products. The ovo-lactovegetarian (or lacto-ovovegetarian) diet also includes eggs. Semi-vegetarians do not eat red meat but include chicken and fish with plant foods, dairy products, and eggs.

Vigorous Physical Activity—Any activity that burns more than 7 kcal/min or the equivalent of 6 or more metabolic equivalents (METs) and results in achieving 74 to 88 percent of peak heart rate. An estimate of a person's peak heart rate can be obtained by subtracting the person's age from 220. Examples of vigorous physical activity include jogging, mowing the lawn with a nonmotorized push mower, chopping wood, participating in high-impact aerobic dancing, swimming continuous laps, or bicycling uphill. Vigorous-intensity physical activity may be intense enough to represent a substantial challenge to an individual and results in a significant increase in heart and breathing rate.

Weight-Bearing Exercise—Any activity one performs that works bones and muscles against gravity, including walking, running, hiking, dancing, gymnastics, and soccer.

Whole Grains—Foods made from the entire grain seed, usually called the kernel, which consists of the bran, germ, and endosperm. If the kernel has been cracked, crushed, or flaked, it must retain nearly the same relative proportions of bran, germ, and endosperm as the original grain in order to be called whole grain.[16]

---

[16] AACC Press Release, AACC To Create Consumer-Friendly Whole Grain Definition, March 5, 2004.
http://www.aaccnet.org/news/CFWholeGrain.asp.

APPENDIX D. ACRONYMS

AI–Adequate Intakes
AMDR–Acceptable Macronutrient Distribution Range
ARS–Agricultural Research Service
BMI–Body Mass Index
CSFII–Continuing Survey of Food Intakes by Individuals
DASH–Dietary Approaches to Stop Hypertension
DFE–Dietary Folate Equivalent
DHA–Docosahexaenoic acid
DRI–Dietary Reference Intake
DV–Daily Value
EAR–Estimated Average Requirement
EER–Estimated Energy Requirement
EPA–Eicosapentaenoic acid
FDA–Food and Drug Administration
FDAMA–Food and Drug Administration Modernization Act
HDL–High-density lipoprotein
HHS–U.S. Department of Health and Human Services
IU–International unit
LDL–Low-density lipoprotein
RAE–Retinol Activity Equivalent
RDA–Recommended Dietary Allowance
USDA–U.S. Department of Agriculture

NOTES